Springer Series on Nursing Management and Leadership

Joyce J. Fitzpatrick, PhD, RN, MBA, FAAN, Series Editor

Advisory Board:
Pamela Cipriano, PhD, RN, FAAN; Harriet R. Feldman, PhD, RN, FAAN; Greer Glazer, RN, PhD, CNP, FAAN; Daniel J. Pesut, PhD, APRN, BC, FAAN

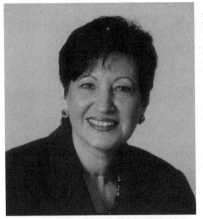

Harriet R. Feldman, PhD, RN, FAAN, is Dean and Professor at the Lienhard School of Nursing and Chair of the Institutional Review Board at Pace University. She is the Editor of the journal *Nursing Leadership Forum*. Dr. Feldman has authored more than 60 articles, book chapters, and editorials, is co-author of *Nurses in the Political Arena: The Public Face of Nursing,* and editor of *Strategies for Nursing Leadership* and *Nursing Leaders Speak Out: Issues and Opinions.* She has served in leadership roles in a number of professional organizations, including the New York State Nurses Association, the American Association of Colleges of Nursing, Sigma Theta Tau International, Nurses Educational Fund, and on the boards of the Commission on Collegiate Nursing Education and Nyack Hospital.

The
Nursing Shortage

Strategies for Recruitment and Retention in Clinical Practice and Education

Harriet R. Feldman, PhD, RN, FAAN
Editor

 Springer Publishing Company

Copyright © 2003 Springer Publishing Company, Inc.

Springer Publishing Company, Inc.
536 Broadway
New York, NY 10012-3955

Acquisitions Editor: Ruth Chasek
Production Editor: Jean Hurkin-Torres
Cover design by Joanne Honigman

03 04 05 06 07 / 5 4 3 2 1

Library of Congress Cataloging-in-Publication Data

The nursing shortage : strategies for recruitment and retention in
  clinical practice and education / Harriet Feldman, editor.
     p. ; cm. – (Springer series on nursing management and leadership)
  Includes bibliographical references and index.
  ISBN 0-8261-2165-9
    1. Nursing—Administration. 2. Nurses—Supply and demand.
  3. Manpower planning. 4. Medical personnel—Supply and demand.
  I. Feldman, Harriet R. II. Series.
    [DNLM: 1. Nursing—manpower—United States. WY 16 N978731 2003]
  RT89.N83 2003
  331.12'9161073'0973—dc22

                                 2003057353

Printed in the United States of America by Maple-Vail Manufacturing Group.

Contents

Contributors

Jane Aroian, EdD, RN
Associate Professor
Northeastern University School
  of Nursing
Bowe College of Health Sciences
Boston, MA

Doreen Begley, MS, RN
Nurse Executive
Nevada Hospital Association
Reno, NV

David N. Bennett, PhD, RN
Chair
School of Nursing
Kennesaw State University
Kennesaw, GA

**Suzanne C. Beyea, RN, PhD,
  FAAN**
Director of Research
Association of PeriOperative
  Registered Nurses (AORN)
Denver, CO

Marie N. Bremner, DSN, RN, CS
Associate Professor
Kennesaw State University
Kennesaw, GA

Judith A. Cohen, PhD, RN
Associate Professor
University of Vermont
College of Nursing and Health
  Sciences
Burlington, VT

**Rosanna DeMarco, PhD, RN,
  ACRN**
Assistant Professor
Boston College School of Nursing
Chestnut Hill, MA

Susan W. Devaney, EdD, RN, CS
FIPSE Project Facilitator
Moberly Area Community
  College
Moberly, MO; and
University of Missouri
Sinclair School of Nursing
Columbia, MO

Barbara R. Heller, EdD, RN, FAAN
Executive Director
Center for Health Workforce
  Development
University of Maryland
Baltimore, MD

Christine Henriksen, AAS, RN
Patient Service Leader
University Hospital
SUNY Upstate Medical University
Syracuse, NY

Julie E. Johnson, PhD, RN
Director and Professor
Orvis School of Nursing
University of Nevada, Reno
Reno, NV

Ruth J. Jones, MSN, RN
Director of Allied Health
Moberly Area Community College
Moberly, MO

Ann Marie Kotzer, PhD, RN
Director
Nursing Research
The Children's Hospital; and
Assistant Professor
University of Colorado School of
    Nursing
Denver, CO

**Alice F. Kuehn, PhD, RN, CS,
    FNP/GNP**
Associate Professor
University of Missouri
Sinclair School of Nursing
Columbia, MO

Leslie P. Lichtenberg, BA
President
Trio Communications
Baltimore, MD

Andrea Lindell, DNSc, RN
Dean and Senior Associate Vice
    President
College of Nursing
University of Cincinnati
Cincinnati, OH

Eugenia Mills, MSN, RN
Chairperson
Department of Nursing
Miami University
Miami, FL

Lynne Ott, MSN, RN
Director of Nursing
Fitzgibbon Hospital
Marshall, MO

**Nancy E. Page, MS, APRN, BC-
    ADM, CDE**
Coordinator of Nursing Practice
University Hospital
SUNY Upstate Medical University
Syracuse, NY

Mary Val Palumbo, MSN, APRN
University of Vermont
College of Nursing and Health
    Sciences
Burlington, VT

Nancy Polatty, MS, RN, JD
Assistant Professor
Orvis School of Nursing
University of Nevada, Reno
Reno, NV

Bonnie Raingruber, PhD, RN
Professor of Nursing
California State University; and
Nurse Researcher
Center for Nursing Research
University of California–Davis
Sacramento, CA

Betty Rambur, DNSc, RN
Dean and Professor
University of Vermont
College of Nursing and Health
    Sciences
Burlington, VT

Victoria Ritter, RN, MBA
Nurse Manager
University of California Davis
  Medical Center
Sacramento, CA

Susan Schmidt, PhD, RN
Chairperson
Department of Nursing
Xavier University
Cincinnati, OH

Thomas Shaw, PhD
Research Associate
Institute for Policy Research
University of Cincinnati
Cincinnati, OH

Hrafn Óli Sigurðsson, PhD, RN, CNOR
Resident Consultant/Advisor
Nursing Development Office
Landspítali University Hospital
Reykjavik, Iceland

Gail Smart, MS, RN
Nursing Recruitment and
  Retention
The Children's Hospital
Denver, CO

Richard K. Sowell, PhD, RN, FAAN
Dean, College of Health and
  Human Services
Kennesaw State University
Kennesaw, GA

Carolyn Thomas, MSN, RN
Vice President for Patient Care
  Services, Chief Nursing Officer
The University Hospital
Cincinnati, OH

Joan Trofino, EdD, CNAA, FAAN
Associate Professor
Department of Nursing
University of Nevada
Las Vegas, NV

Alfred Tuchfarber, PhD
Director
Institute for Policy Research
University of Cincinnati
Cincinnati, OH

Darla Vale, DNSc, RN
Chairperson
Department of Health Sciences
College of Mount St. Joseph
Cincinnati, OH

Richard Williams II, AAS, RN
Patient Service Leader
University Hospital
SUNY Upstate Medical University
Syracuse, NY

Priscilla Sandford Worral, PhD, RN
Coordinator for Nursing
  Research
University Hospital
SUNY Upstate Medical University
Syracuse, NY

Preface

The shortage of nurses in the United States is moving toward crisis proportions. Although most schools of nursing have seen increases in enrollments in the recent past, the numbers being prepared for the workforce are nowhere near what is needed now and in the immediate and long-term future. Because of a parallel shortage of qualified nursing faculty, many schools are unable to accept additional students, although waiting lists are common for these institutions. Unless we find innovative and creative ways to ameliorate the shortage, it will continue to grow. Short-term initiatives, such as accelerated baccalaureate nursing programs for non-nurse career change prospects, are growing nationally. Longer-term strategies include image campaigns and outreach to elementary- and middle-school children. We need also to provide appropriate graduate education in nursing to prepare the faculty leaders of tomorrow and to retain the current workforce.

The Nursing Shortage: Strategies for Recruitment and Retention in Clinical Practice and Education focuses on what communities, organizations, and individuals are doing to address the nursing shortage. A call for papers for a special issue of *Nursing Leadership Forum* was sent to nursing leaders based on a conversation I had with deans of nursing education programs about their efforts to work collaboratively with their nursing service partners to expand the workforce of baccalaureate-prepared nurses. The call yielded a diverse array of papers from many sectors that offer creative opportunities for us to consider. Among the strategies described are service and education models for partnering, joint appointments, joint collaboration in research, succession planning, preceptor and mentoring arrangements, scholarships and work payback agreements, and private and public funding initiatives to support the education of future nurses.

The first three chapters approach the topic from a statewide perspective in Vermont (Cohen, Palumbo, and Rambur), Missouri (Devaney, Kuehn, Jones, and Ott), and Nevada (Johnson, Polatty, and Begley). The fourth chapter, authored by Beyea, provides the perspective of a national specialty organization, the Association of PeriOperative Registered Nurses (AORN), to recruit and retain nurses in the area of OR nursing. These four chapters comprise Part I: The Policy Front. The four articles that follow comprise Part II: The Education Front, and describe educational partnerships with service, private foundations and corporations, and government, representing initiatives in the states of Maryland (Heller and Lichtenberg), Georgia (Bennett, Bremner, and Sowell), and Massachusetts (DeMarco and Aroian), and the City of Cincinnati, Ohio (Vale, Schmidt, Mills, Shaw, Lindell, Thomas, and Tuchfarber). Part III: The Retention Front has five chapters. The first four focus on the work setting in terms of recruitment and retention, with chapters that consider an urban emergency room (Raingruber and Ritter), power sharing (Trofino), a tertiary care pediatric setting (Smart and Kotzer), and the recruitment/retention challenges in a major medical center (Henriksen, Williams, Page, and Worral). The last chapter adds an international perspective, with the focus on a retention effort in Iceland.

As the 13 chapters convey, we must all be part of the solution. I believe that the ideas presented are worthy of application to other settings, and hope that you will seriously consider them as opportunities for your work setting to make changes that support and grow the nursing workforce.

HARRIET R. FELDMAN, PHD, RN, FAAN
EDITOR

PART ONE

The Policy Front

CHAPTER ONE

Combating the Nursing Shortage: Vermont's Call to Action

Judith A. Cohen, Mary Val Palumbo, and Betty Rambur

Vermont is known for its natural beauty and high quality of life, yet it is not immune to the national issues and problems that pervade our society. Vermont, like the rest of the nation, is experiencing a nursing shortage, which, if not corrected, will negatively impact the health and quality of life of Vermonters.

National studies and reports have identified factors that have led to a profound nursing shortage: the aging of society (Martin et al., 2001); an aging nursing workforce (Buerhaus, Staiger, & Auerbach, 2000a; Minnick, 2000); a decline in nursing enrollments (American Association of Colleges or Nursing [AACN], 2001; Nevidjon & Erikson, 2001); increasing technology and other advances (Aiken, 1995; Buerhaus, Staiger, & Auerbach, 2000b), and a shrinking pool of qualified nursing faculty (Sloane, 1999). This shortage is uniquely serious in that it is connected to both an increased demand for, and also a decreased supply of nurses. The demand for nursing services is particularly related to the expected doubling of the elder population by 2030 as the baby boom generation ages, while the number of women aged 25–54, who have traditionally formed the core of the nursing workforce, will remain unchanged. By 2020, 1.75 million more registered nurses will be needed, but if current trends continue only 635,000 will be available. The high national nursing vacancy rate of 11% in hospitals and even higher rates in extended care facilities attest to the supply factors leading to the nursing shortage, particularly job dissatisfaction related to difficult existing work conditions and stagnant nursing salaries.

This chapter describes the centrality of the nursing leadership role in Vermont's statewide efforts to combat the nursing shortage, particularly the establishment of a Blue Ribbon Commission and an Office of Nursing Workforce Research, Planning, and Development. These efforts have been cumulative, characterized by innovation and unprecedented collaboration between stakeholders representing nursing, public health, health care administration, education, and the political and private sectors.

DEVELOPMENT OF THE BLUE RIBBON COMMISSION

The development of the Blue Ribbon Commission was preceded by initial work done by the Vermont Organization of Nurse Leaders (VONL), a member of the Coalition of Vermont Nursing Organizations (COVNO), which "provides leadership, professional development and networking opportunities in order to advance patient and health care delivery, promote excellence in nursing leadership, develop and maximize systems in which professional nurses practice, and influence health policy"(Kaeding, 1998). This foundational work was essential in creating a climate for change. Highlights are as follows.

In 1998, the VONL, in conjunction with the Vermont Association of Hospital and Health Systems (VAHHS), commissioned a report to evaluate the state of nursing in Vermont and its impact on hospitals. Information was obtained through surveys that were distributed to hospitals and health systems, with return rates of 100% from hospitals, 30% from home health agencies, and a small number from long-term care. *The Report on Nursing* (Kaeding, 1998) identified four trends within the state that are similar to national trends: an aging population of current registered nurses, a diminishing number of new nursing students entering the profession (36%), an increase in the utilization of nurses in all parts of the health care sector, and stagnation of wages for nurses.

The Vermont Organization of Nurse Leaders, in conjunction with VAHHS, hosted the first statewide Nursing Summit in November 1999 in which more than 100 stakeholders came together to discuss the state of nursing in Vermont. At the summit they began to identify solutions and time frames for action. A variety of nursing leadership organizations were represented, including the VONL, the Vermont State

Nurses Association (VSNA), Kappa Tau Chapter of Sigma Theta Tau International, and representatives from public health, health care administration, education, and political and public sectors. The discussion focused on information presented in the prior year's *Report on Nursing* in Vermont (Kaeding, 1998) and began to identify ways to broaden the data contained within the report to include the state of nursing in community and long-term-care settings. Work groups were formed, with members from each constituency focused on the challenges for educational institutions and barriers to education, recruitment and retention issues within the profession and in clinical settings, workplace practice issues, and the changing health care environment and public policy issues.

Following the summit in the summer of 2000, members of the VONL presented the *Report on Nursing* in Vermont (Kaeding, 1998) and the work of the summit group (VONL, 2000a) with recommendations to the Public Oversight Commission (POC), a state regulatory agency charged to control health care costs. The presentation provided a status report on the nursing workforce and outlined concerns related to hospital functioning and budgets. The presentation emphasized that research has established the relationship between the presence and availability of registered nurses and quality of care (Kavner & Gergen, 1998), yet supply has been insufficient and based on current trends would be increasingly insufficient in the future. Moreover, the presentation emphasized that registered nurses in Vermont are the most rapidly aging group, largely secondary to a concomitantly smaller cohort of younger nurses; the average RN age was 46, with 75% over

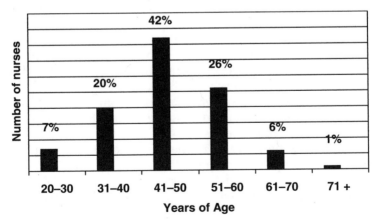

FIGURE 1.1 Age of RN's Working in Vermont.

40 years of age (see Figure 1.1). The presentation also illustrated trend data to clarify that RN wages were not only flat when adjusted for inflation, but also that the average starting salaries for nursing graduates fell 3.4% from 1997–1998 when compared to other college graduates. Based upon data collection done annually by VAHHS and summarized in their January 2000 vacancy data, the presentation indicated that the overall vacancy rate for registered nurses was 7.4%, for licensed practical nurses, 11.3%, and for licensed nursing assistants, 13.3%. Consequently, as vacancies increased, hospital salary and benefit costs rose as a result of (a) increased use of traveling nurses; (b) increased overtime; (c) incentives required for working extra shifts; (d) increased recruitments costs from sign-on bonuses and training costs; and (e) increased costs for retention. The data were of particular concern to the POC, given their responsibility to control the extent to which hospital budgets can increase. Finally, the impact of the nursing shortage on public health was presented to the POC, including the potential for decreased quality of care, increased length of patient stay in hospitals due to lack of staffing in tertiary care and nursing homes, intermittent closing of beds and transfer of patients to other hospitals, and loss of public confidence in local health care institutions.

An updated report (VONL, 2000b), *The Current State of Nursing in Vermont,* then encapsulated *The Report on Nursing in Vermont* (Kaeding, 1998), identified some solutions, and described a beginning strategic plan generated at the summit meeting to reverse the shortage and strengthen Vermont nursing. The first recommendation of this report was to create a Blue Ribbon Panel representative of nursing and community leaders. The panel was envisioned to develop the strategies outlined in the report and detail an action plan by the end of 2000. As envisioned, their activities were to include

1. utilizing current resources within VONL, the Vermont State Nurses Association, and specialty organizations to promote positive support for practicing Vermont nurses;

2. utilizing human-resource associations within VAHHS to analyze wage structures and recommend salary and benefits changes necessary to attract and retain nurses;

3. disseminating the contents of the report to all CEOs and CFOs in institutions across the continuum with nursing systems;

4. obtaining POC approval for increased dollars and FTEs within hospital budgets to implement necessary nursing initiatives (VONL, 2000b).

This recommendation received immediate public and high-level support. Specifically, Jane Kitchel, Vermont's Secretary of Human Services, capitalized on the momentum and established the Blue-Ribbon Commission during the summer of 2000. The Commission was thus charged to "develop recommendations that can be used by public policy makers, educators and providers, to ensure an adequate nursing work force to meet the health care needs of Vermont" (Blue Ribbon Commission, 2001, p. 1). The Commission, chaired by Dr. Robert Clarke, chancellor of the Vermont state colleges, was bold in its breadth and diversity, with 27 members again representing a broad-based constituency in both the private and public sectors. Much of the membership was drawn from those who attended the nursing summit.[1]

The tone for success was set in the first meeting, when a compelling overview of need was detailed, followed by a summary of the efforts to date. An ambitious and firm timeline was set, with meetings every 3 weeks and the expectation of a final product in 16 weeks. National articles and research were distributed to commission members to assure baseline knowledge for deliberations. It was also emphasized that the Blue Ribbon Commission was to build upon the previous efforts without reinventing the wheel.

PROCESS FOR THE BLUE RIBBON COMMISSION

Early on Edward Connors[2] provided broad process points upon which to guide the deliberations (Figure 1.2). The Commission then divided into several committees to accomplish its goals: prioritization committee, research committee, education committee, nursing practice environment committee, and committee on partnerships for success. The prioritization committee was designed to help focus the numerous issues discussed. A research subcommittee was charged with coordinating data collection from numerous resources and reports.[3] The remaining committees were established to focus on three areas of concentration within the report: education, nursing practice environment, and partnerships for success. Each of these committees was charged to focus on the strengths, weaknesses, opportunities, and threats as well as to identify short- and long-term strategies to deal with the opportunities and threats. The committees reported back to the whole commission every 3 weeks.

FIGURE 1.2 Guidelines for the Blue Ribbon Commission Process

1. Clarify what audience you intend to influence.
2. Focus and limit issues that we intend to address in our recommendations.
3. Begin early to conceptualize our final report in both the structure and content. Assign responsibility for drafting early conclusions and recommendations facilitating focused debate and resolution.
4. Accept the reality that many issues and interests have insufficient data for our purposes.
5. Rely on the judgment and experience of the panel members, focusing on group consensus.
6. Accept the reality that there is no quick fix or silver bullet because these are complex issues.
7. Consider in the report the context of the long-term view. Have a set of directions, not solutions. Articulate a few immediate steps with much specificity but develop a long-term vision.
8. Develop a realistic plan for the dissemination and follow-up on report recommendations, including building support and understanding, exciting stakeholders.
9. Educational preparation does make a positive difference. RN mix in acute hospitals can make a difference.
10. Tackle the issues of what it will take to improve environments where nursing services are provided, with an emphasis on quality patient care and urging stakeholders to turn to meaningful collaboration to solve the Vermont challenges. Identify what attributes are in place in effective institutions.
11. Conclusions and recommendations will cover increase supply, educational preparation, retention, work environment, collaboration. Put in context of a doable plan and refine national conclusions for Vermont.

Source note: Minutes of August 21, 2000 meeting, Blue Ribbon Commission, Vermont State Colleges, Waterbury, Vermont.

FACTORS AND ISSUES AFFECTING THE STATE OF NURSING IN VERMONT

Seventeen issues and challenges were identified (Figure 1.3). These were collapsed by the Commission into seven problem statements (Table 1.1): the changing health care environment; inaccurate public perceptions; barriers to education; underutilization of partnerships;

FIGURE 1.3 Blue Ribbon Commission Issues/Factors Affecting the Nursing Shortage.

1. Structural problems
2. K–12 linkages
3. Public relations/image of nursing
4. Technology
5. Retention
6. Higher-education issues
7. Gender issues/diversity issues
8. "Value of nursing" issues
9. Changing health care system
10. Quality of care
11. Developing partnerships
12. Why is this a "profession in crisis"?
13. Setting the public policy agenda
14. Overcoming the cycles of shortages
15. American Nursing Credentialing Center initiative
16. Age of nursing profession
17. All fields/areas of nursing

structural impediments; profession not valued; and issues important to nurses that are not being addressed.

These problem areas identified were further collapsed into the factors that appeared in the *Report and Recommendations of the Blue Ribbon Commission*. Some of them were focused for immediate action, such as improving the workplace environment, increasing nursing education capacity and decreasing barriers to education, increasing recruitment and retention of nurses in the practice setting, changing public perception of nursing as a career, and enhancing partnerships and salary structures. Others, though interlinked with the above, were targeted for focused action in the future. These include continuing to improve conditions in the workplace, enhancing collaborative relationships between physicians and nurses, and developing the workforce of other health care personnel. The Commission's recommendations were specifically targeted to the factors that decrease the supply of nurses, increase the demand on nurses, and create high stress environments in the workplace (Table 1.2). The Blue Ribbon Commission (2001) issued a call to action to address the nursing shortage in Vermont through seven recommendations found in Figure 1.4. What follows is a description of progress on these recommendations.

TABLE 1.1 Problem Areas Affecting the State of Nursing in Vermont

Problem Areas	Defining Characteristics
Changing health care environment (Increased Demand on Nurses)	Burdensome federal and state regulatory requirements
	Agency budget cuts and inadequate federal reimbursements to agencies
	Insularity of nurses from national "system" issues
	Redesigning of nursing roles
	Aging of both nurses and the general population
	Higher acuity in hospitals, increased chronic illness
Inaccurate Public Perception of Nursing	Nursing role being ill defined or understood
	Variety of career opportunities in nursing not emphasized
	Medical errors and publicity
	Mostly female profession
	Perceptions of career by counselors, parents, others
	Nurses often degrading own profession
	Relationship of quality measures and nursing not understood.
Barriers to Nursing Education	Personal and institutional budget constraints, costs
	Availability of loans/scholarships, tuition reimbursement, work release time, advanced degree certification education, reentry opportunities, clinical experience, distance education opportunities for adult learners
	Fewer faculty, school closings

(continued)

TABLE 1.1 (*continued*)

Problem Areas	Defining Characteristics
Underutilization of partnerships	Providers, nursing schools, and K–12 grades
	Limited collaboration between/with professional boards, associations, higher education, state government, and physicians
	Limited number of nurse leaders to create local/regional/state collaborations
	Underutilization of multidisciplinary models
Structural Impediments	Same licensure examination for all entry level of education
	Federal requirements for documentation and examination
	Less management support
	Compressed pay scale for skills and education
	Low pay and benefits
	Shift work
	Lack of understanding about how to utilize aging nurses
	Burnout
	A change in work ethic
	Insurance gatekeeping that prevents access to nurses in advanced practice
Perception of the profession not being valued	Nurses degrading their own profession
	Poor nurse-physician relationships

(*continued*)

TABLE 1.1 (*continued*)

Problem Areas	Defining Characteristics
	Feelings of lack of empowerment and not being a part of the decision-making team
	Therapeutic input is not documented or valued
	Science of nursing not fully recognized
	Impact on quality of care that nursing provides is not well known or documented
	Technology not a priority to assist in management or documentation
	Salary structure does not reflect value of nursing
Important issues to nursing which were not seen as being addressed	Workplace safety, needlestick legislation
Important issues to nursing which were not seen as being addressed	Mandatory overtime
	Staff and patient mix
	Direct care nurse's involvement in decision on staffing levels
	Whistle-blower protection
	Appropriate utilization of nurses
	Salary/benefits
	Stressful workplace environments

Source note: Office of nursing workforce (2002). Registered Nurses in Vermont. Retrieved from *http://www.choosenursingvermont.org.*

TABLE 1.2 Factors Targeted by the Blue Ribbon Commission Recommendations

Facts Leading to Nursing Shortage	Contributing Factors/Conditions
Decreased supply	Fewer students entering nursing education programs
	Aging nursing workforce
	More nursing time spent on administrative duties
Increased demand	Increased utilization of nurses
	Increased training in information and technology
	Additional nursing administrative duties
High-stress workplace environment	Shortages/reduced workforce leading to burnout
	Hazardous work environments

Source note: Minutes of August 21, 2000 meetings Blue Ribbon Commission, Vermont State Colleges, Waterbury, Vermont.

PROGRESS TO DATE ON THE BLUE RIBBON COMMISSION RECOMMENDATIONS

CREATE A CENTER FOR NURSING

To aid in the development of a Center for Nursing, an advisory board[4] was formed. By December 2001, the advisory board chose a manager of the Office of Nursing Workforce, Research, Planning, and Development and the work of the office was begun. The University of Vermont has a specific definition of the term *center* and stipulates that it must be a multidisciplinary, self-supporting entity. An adjustment to the name was therefore needed to better reflect the specific functions of this new entity. These functions include: a) designing, conducting, and reporting the research on the nature of the nursing workforce in Vermont; b) communicating and collaborating with the state college system, Agency of Human Services, University of Vermont, Area Health

FIGURE 1.4 Blue Ribbon Commission Recommendations.
January 2001

1. Create a Center for Nursing located at the University of Vermont
   in collaboration with the Vermont state Colleges to address
   ongoing issues of supply, education, practice, and research
   (annual cost: $250,000).
2. Form a state-funded Vermont Nursing Education Loan Forgiveness
   Program (loan forgivenessness would be linked to an agreement to
   practice nursing in Vermont for a specified period of time) (annual
   cost: $400,000).
3. Develop an aggressive fundraising effort to raise scholarship
   support for nursing students from private sources.
4. Establish a partnership between the state of Vermont, health care
   providers, educators, and other health care partners to promote
   the profession of nursing (annual cost $250,000).
5. Increase state funding to expand nursing continuing-education
   programs. This include a) funding to create a virtual continuing
   education organization for nurses in all organizational settings.
   Activities would include a comprehensive assessment of learning
   needs as well as program implementation; b) development of more
   short-term courses via distance learning for working nurses; and
   c) development of courses to prepare nurses to practice in
   specialized settings such as critical care, operating room, and
   mental health (annual cost: $350,000).
6. Expand the capacity of existing nursing education programs so
   that they can prepare more students (annual cost: $500,000).
7. Increase nursing salaries to retain nurses and attract new nurses
   into the profession.

The recommendations were submitted for comment via public
hearings during November and December. These hearings were
conducted at a number of Vermont Interactive Television sites
throughout the state to ensure wide public access and members of
the commission were present at each of these hearings. The Blue
Ribbon Commission Report was finalized in December and was
released and disseminated via a public press conference at the
Vermont State House in Montpelier, Vermont, on January 25, 2001.

Education Center (AHEC), and health care providers regarding the
Vermont nursing workforce; c) securing grant funding for the long-
term viability of the office; and d) coordinating with other statewide
initiatives such as the Freeman Nurse Scholars Program and the Student Loan Forgiveness Program (both described later).

Start-up funding ($95,000) for the first year came from the Agency of Human Services. An HRSA Rural Health Outreach grant ($347,000) was received by June 2002. A third grant from the Federal Office of Rural Health Policy ($50,000) was also obtained during the first year. Total funding ($492,000) made it possible to create an ambitious research, education, and practice agenda. The manager of the Office of Nursing Workforce is responsible for the allocation of these funds with the input of nurse researchers, clinicians, and educators as well as policy makers and stakeholders throughout the state. The three primary agendas of the office follow.

1. A *research agenda* was set with the purpose of getting accurate information about the status of Vermont's nursing workforce to all stakeholders as quickly as possible. The relicensure surveys for RNs, LPNs and LNAs used by the State Board of Nursing and analyzed by the Health Department were chosen for secondary analysis and redesign. Previous relicensure studies were not done on a regular basis and the data collected were not comprehensively reviewed. Data regarding "intention to leave" a primary position was particularly important to understand in order to predict future supply needs (Figure 1.5). Replacement of the biannual "vacancy rate" survey was also identified as a pressing need. The vacancy rate survey of hospitals, extended care facilities, and home health agencies had been done for 13 years and was eliminated by its sponsoring agency as of February 2001. A research team consisting of faculty from biometry, nursing,

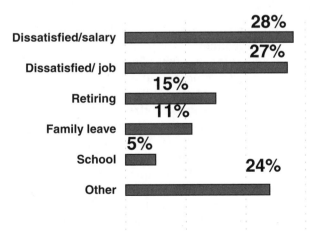

FIGURE 1.5 Data from 2001 RN Relicensure Survey, Likeliness to Leave Primary Position

business, and economics was formed to develop a more accurate tool for assessment of the demand for Vermont's health care workers.

The older nurse was chosen as another focus for investigation because 75% of Vermont's nurses are over age 40. Management practices, job characteristics, and choice of settings, as well as physical and emotional issues for this population of nurses (age 50+) are being studied by researchers from the college of nursing and business administration. The overall goal is to develop strategies to retain the older worker in nursing, including successful strategies from other industries that may be translated to nursing.

In the long-term-care setting, attempts to find the best practice sites in the state will be made. Staff turnover rate and resident satisfaction data collected by the Office on Aging and Disabilities will guide the investigation to locate and describe examples of innovative workplace practices and culture. A team of nursing executives from the state's long-term care facilities has been assembled for this project.

The middle-school student was chosen as the focus of investigation regarding the perception of an ideal career versus a career in nursing. This study is a replication of a previous study (1991) conducted in Illinois. The convenience sample has been obtained during the summer outreach events in rural areas throughout Vermont. This information will help guide the advertising campaign targeting middle-school students that is planned.

The status of Vermont's reentry programs for RNs with lapsed licenses will also be investigated and described. The numbers of Vermont nurses desiring a reentry program is unknown. The most effective way of conducting a program that prepares nurses for practice in a variety of settings must also be determined. An annual dean's survey that assesses capacity for incoming nursing students as well nursing faculty recruitment and retention will also contribute to the assessment of Vermont's ability to educate nurses.

2. The *educational agenda* of the Office of Nursing Workforce required the hiring of a statewide nurse outreach team. The first assignment for the team was "Choose Nursing Vermont," an exhibition tour of five county fairs or field days. These fairs are all held in rural areas and traditionally attract an agricultural crowd. The flexibility of combining a nursing career and farming is appealing to many in this population. During the school year, the outreach team will make contacts with teachers, school nurses, and guidance counselors in order to have opportunities for presentations to middle-school students about careers in nursing. Efforts will also be made to reach out to Vermont's Native American population, the Abenaki, to boys, and to displaced workers. Minority recruitment is planned by collabora-

tion with the University of Vermont's recruitment efforts in an inner-city high school.

Successful recruiting efforts will challenge Vermont's five schools of nursing to be prepared to accommodate more students. The Office of Nursing Workforce will facilitate dialogue between service and education. Joint faculty appointments and increased opportunities for master's and doctoral studies in a distance education format are desired outcomes. Preceptors involved in the Vermont Nurse Internship program will be the first group targeted for recruitment into master's programs.

3. The *practice agenda* of the Office of Nursing Workforce is in the early stages and will focus on workplace issues of improving patient safety and working conditions. Dialogue about salaries will be facilitated with appropriate stakeholders as opportunities arise. Evidence-based recommendations to retain older workers will be disseminated. Summaries of the research findings from the Office of Nursing Workforce will help direct policy makers and nursing leaders to focus practice initiatives appropriately.

VERMONT NURSING EDUCATION LOAN FORGIVENESS/ LOAN REPAYMENT PROGRAM

For the last 2 years, the Vermont General Assembly passed legislation ensuring nursing loan forgiveness (for students in RN and LPN programs in Vermont) and loan repayment (for working nurses), with $180,000 allocated for fiscal year 2002; $100,000 was designated for the loan repayment program. Loan repayment is available to both RNs and LPNs. The number of applicants for last year was 57, with 21 awards being made (up to $6,000 per nurse); $80,000 was allocated to the loan forgiveness program. Loan forgiveness is available to nursing students in accredited LPN or RN programs. Initially, there were 50 applicants for loan forgiveness, with 13 awards given of $6,000 each. There is a time commitment to work in Vermont in exchange for each of these programs.

RAISE SCHOLARSHIP SUPPORT FOR NURSING STUDENTS FROM PRIVATE SOURCES

The Freeman Nurse Scholars Program was developed through a $3 million contribution from the Stowe–based Freeman Foundation. This program has enhanced the attractiveness of nursing as a career for excellent candidates who agree to practice in the state of Vermont for 2 years after graduation. This merit-based scholarship provides up to

$15,000 for associate-degree scholars and $30,000 for bachelor-degree students. This program represents in-state philanthropy that appears to have stimulated interest in the choice of nursing, as evidenced by increased applications to 4 out of 5 schools and a significant increase in SAT scores at the state's largest program. The duration of this program is 5 years, from 2000 to 2005, with 100 awards of $7,500 made to date out of a total amount of 370 awards.

ESTABLISH A PARTNERSHIP TO PROMOTE THE PROFESSION OF NURSING

The Office of Nursing Workforce has taken the lead in initiating an advertising campaign to promote the image of nursing to Vermont's youth. The first year of the campaign targets middle-school students and is guided by the findings of the research initiative on the image of nursing among middle-school youth described herein. Materials developed by other state initiatives and national organizations will be utilized whenever possible, yet Vermont is a small, rural state and any materials used need to be recognizable by Vermont's youth. Consistency and accuracy of information can be achieved by directing marketing resources through a center office such as Vermont's Office of Nursing Workforce. Radio and television ads, press kits, information packets, Web sites, toll-free numbers, posters, and promotion items will be the communication vehicles for the advertising campaign. Future target audiences will be high-school students, college age students, mothers returning to the workforce, and displaced workers.

Other initiatives that reflect this partnership between the state of Vermont, health care providers, educators, and other health care partners to promote nursing have included the Area Health Education Center (AHEC) Career Pathways Consortium of hospitals, high schools, and technical centers. Mentorship programs with Southern Vermont Technical Centers, summer camps such as the MedQuest Camps, and the Stafford Health Career Academy are all products of such efforts. AHEC has also produced and distributed a Health Careers Resource Book and has provided seed money for the Vermont Nursing Internship Project—a collaboration between VONL/deans and directors of Vermont schools of nursing and hospitals within the state—and Daring to Care, among other programs.

INCREASE STATE FUNDING TO EXPAND NURSING CONTINUING EDUCATION PROGRAMS

A comprehensive assessment of learning needs as well as program implementation was recommended. This assessment has been done informally and more short-term courses via distance learning for working nurses were identified. Regarding the shortage of specialty nurses, Senator Patrick Leahy described Vermont's unique approach to the Senate Judiciary Committee, Immigration Subcommittee as follows:

> Vermont has also addressed its nursing shortage through the use of fees paid by employers using the H-1B program, the visa program for highly skilled temporary workers. Vermont's Department of Employment and Training (DET), on behalf of the Human Resources Investment Council, received $2.7 million in H-1B funds from the U.S. Department of Labor, part of which is being used to implement a health care training program to increase the number of nurses. About 148 specialty nurses in Critical Care and Operating Room nursing have been trained through these funds. The next program will include psychiatric nursing. This is the sort of program that fulfills the promise of our H-1B program—to solve today's worker shortages in a way that will allow us to better fill our own employment needs in the future. (Leahy, 2001)

The Vermont Nurse Internship Program (Boyer, 2002) has addressed the needs of new graduate nurses' transition into the workplace. The mission of this program is to create a formal and sustainable nurse internship program that provides the clinical experience necessary to support the novice's entry into practice, his or her growth along the continuum of expertise, and his or her professional practice within the complex and demanding field of health care. The Vermont Board of Nursing, schools of nursing, and practice sites work in a collaborative, statewide partnership to maintain a nationally recognized Nurse Internship Program. The internship is available in multiple settings and supports the transition from new graduate nurse to a self-confident, adaptable, and independent professional.

Expand the Capacity of Existing Nursing Education

In the time since the Blue Ribbon Commission's recommendations, capacity has been increased at all levels of nursing education. The part-time LPN program has expanded to five sites around the state in conjunction with the Community College of Vermont. This program articulates with the Vermont Technical College associate-degree program, available at four sites. Three other associate degree programs are available due to the expansion of one to a northern site in the last 2 years. Enrollments in 2001 were up 21%. Applications for fall 2002 were up in all five schools of nursing, with increases ranging from 8% to 74%. The University of Vermont has increased its capacity by adding new faculty. Enrollment in the department of nursing has increased

24% at the university in the last 2 years after an unprecedented 74% increase in applications over the previous year. In the future, the Office of Nursing Workforce hopes to be able to recommend an appropriate number of nursing students across the state to meet emerging needs.

INCREASE NURSING SALARIES

Little substantial progress has been made in this area. In a brief survey, six hospitals gave raises in 2001 ranging from 3.5% to 12%, with an average raise of 7.2%. Complex factors associated with reimbursement for health care services, unionization, salary compression, and capital hospital expenditures have impeded the changing of salary structure. Yet millions of dollars are paid to traveling nurses at all hospitals in the state. The cost of replacing a nurse has been calculated to be as high as $20,000. The Senate Committee on Health and Human Services has suggested the formation of a second blue ribbon commission after hearing testimony on the nursing shortage in the spring of 2002. Ongoing forums for meaningful discussion are needed to address this issue and the challenge of improving the work environment of Vermont's nurse workforce. A symposium for hospital CEOs and nurse leaders was planned for November 2002 with the hopes of beginning a statewide dialogue on improving nurses' salaries and working conditions, as well as to forge new partnerships between education and practice, including innovative practitioner-teacher models. To date, such models have been thwarted by logistics stemming from the rural nature of the state and, more disconcerting, by bureaucracy in both education and practice.

CONCLUSION

Vermont has taken its first steps to address its looming nursing shortage. The size of the state, both in terms of population and geography, makes Vermont an ideal laboratory for the incubation of innovative strategies to address the antecedents of the nursing shortage. The size of the state also facilitates systematic evaluation of the consequences of such innovation. Sound evaluation requires reliable and valid data collected over an extended period of time. Moreover, comprehensive evaluation demands these data from a diversity of sources using multiple methods. Finally, these data must be disseminated in a manner that can inform stakeholders and guide further policy formation.

The structure for accomplishing change now exists in Vermont. The Vermont experience offers important lessons for other states or regions desiring to undertake such action (Table 1.3). In the final analysis, however, this nursing initiative will only be deemed successful if safe, effective nursing care can be delivered by well-compensated professionals. Appropriate compensation will necessarily impact overall health-care expenditures, with a corollary impact on health-care financing, budgeting, and revenue generation. Because the revenue for health services is ultimately drawn from taxes in the case of Medicare, Medicaid, and Tricare, employers and employees through employer-based insurance premiums, and individuals through out-of-pocket expenses, a broader and deeper public understanding of the interrela-

TABLE 1.3 Lessons Learned

Context is important.	Understand the political, social, and economic environment.
	Build upon what has been done.
	Engage and impassion a broad range of public and private sector stakeholders from both within and outside of higher education, public policy, and healthcare.
Gather firm data, move swiftly and decisively.	Set and achieve firm deadlines and expectations.
	Progress builds confidence. Confidence brings momentum. Momentum mounts excitement. Excitement catalyzes visibility. Visibility expands opportunity.
Court unlikely or unexpected partners	Establish collaborative relationships with philanthropy, the business community, and the press.
	Reconcile historic "competitors" (such as nursing programs in different systems or under different ownership) through innovative, novel, and highly public collaborations.
	Maintain visibility by keeping stakeholders informed.

tionship among nursing salaries, recruitment and retention of nurses, and quality of health care is essential. This is particularly critical in light of the current economic downturn. Individuals, employers, and the government are facing increasing demands for scarce resources. Consequently, health-care facilities will be forced to prioritize their spending in a manner that recognizes the foundational role nurses play in achieving high-quality care. Evidence suggests this will require a substantial reordering of priorities and perceptions within many provider organizations. Nevertheless, public demand for safe, high-quality care is likely to accelerate, as is public recognition of nurses' pivotal role in achieving this outcome.

Nurses conduct a major portion of the overall work of health-care and constitute a proportionally large number of providers within the overall health system. Efforts directed at the nursing workforce are therefore an important and necessary first step. The multifaceted nature of health, however, renders this initiative incomplete without parallel efforts to address the interconnections among health services and the corresponding array of disciplines that provide these services. Similar efforts are needed to expand Vermont's nursing initiative to include allied health professionals and paraprofessionals. Vermont's experience suggests that the social climate is conducive to developing new collaborations and unexpected partnerships. Nevertheless, sustained efforts are needed to assure adequate numbers of nurses and other providers in the foreseeable future. In 10 years, the results of today's efforts will be apparent and will be judged to be visionary, adequate, or shortsighted. It therefore behooves us all to create a world in which we are willing to live.

FOOTNOTES

1. Membership of the Blue Ribbon Commission included the deans, directors, and faculty of the nursing educational programs in Vermont; leaders of nursing in hospitals, community and public health nursing; leaders of the VONL, Vermont State Nurses Association, Vermont Health Care Association, Vermont Association of Hospitals and Health Systems, the Vermont Recruitment Center; commissioner of the Vermont Department of Health; associate dean of the University of Vermont College of Medicine; two members of the state legislature (one from the House of Representatives and one from the Senate); as well as one board member from one of the local hospitals, a nurse board member of the Board of Commissioners, Joint Commission on Accreditation of Health Care Organizations; and the senior policy advisor, Agency of Human Services.

2. Edward Connors is a prior executive with the Mercy Hospital System and is nationally involved in an Institute of Medicine study on nursing staffing in

hospitals and nursing homes (Wunderlick, Sloane, & Davis, 1996) and in the Secretary's Commission on Nursing in 1988 (U.S. Department of Health and Human Services, 1988).

3. Some of these sources included Vermont State Board of Nursing surveys from 1995 and 1997; State Board of Nursing demographics available for at least the past 10 years; the Kaeding report (1998); the VAHHS Annual Statistic Report and Vacancy Survey of June 2000; the Health Resources and Services Administration: National Sample Survey of Registered Nurses 2000, Health Workforce Personnel Factbook (1996); the VONL Report to the Public Oversight Committee; and the Vermont Schools of Nursing annual report of graduates for 1980, 1990, and 1999. Other data collected were current demographics of enrolled registered nurses, licensed practical nurses (LPNs) and licensed nursing assistants (LNAs) in Vermont, comparing enrollment to the past 10 years, salary of registered nurses based on setting and as compared to regional and national trends, data from all Vermont schools of nursing related to debt on graduation of nursing students and comparing debt to other graduates of similar institutions. Where possible, Vermont data were compared to regional and national data.

4. The advisory board consisted of the following members: two from schools of nursing; the president of Lyndon State College; CEO of Central Vermont Medical Center, CEO emerita of the Copley Health System, CEO of Visiting Nurse Association; senior policy advisor from the Agency of Human Services; and the associate dean for primary care in the University of Vermont College of Medicine and physician director of the Area Health Education Center.

REFERENCES

Aiken, L. H. (1995). Transformation of the nursing workforce. *Nursing Outlook, 43*, 201–209.

American Association of Colleges of Nursing. (2001). Nursing school enrollments continue to post decline, though at a slower rate. Retrieved from *http://www.aacn.nche.edu/Media/NewsReleasesEnrol100.htm.*

Blue Ribbon Commission. (2001). A call to action: Addressing Vermont's nursing shortage. *Report and Recommendations of the Blue Ribbon Commission.*

Boyer, S. (2002). Vermont nurse internship project: A collaborative enterprise developed by nurse leaders from education, practice, and regulation. *Nursing Education Perspectives, 23*(2), 81–85.

Buerhaus, P. I., Staiger, D. O., & Auerbach, D. I. (2000a). Implications of an aging registered workforce. *Journal of the American Medical Association, 238*(22), 2948–2954.

Buerhaus, P. I., Staiger, D. O., & Auerbach, D. I. (2000b). Why are shortages of hospital RN's concentrated in specialty care units? *Nursing Economics, 18*(3), 111–116.

Kaeding, T. (1998). *Report on Nursing in Vermont.* Vermont Organization of Nurse Leaders. Vermont Association of Hospitals and Health Systems,

Montpelier, Vermont. Available online: http://www.vahhs.org/lucie/vonl/vsna%20article.htm.

Kovner, C., & Gergen, P. (1998). Nurse staffing levels and adverse events following surgery in U.S. hospitals. *Image: Journal of Nursing Scholarship, 30*(4), 315–321.

Leahy, P. (2001). Hearing statement on "Immigration Policy: Rural and Urban Health Care Needs" at the Senate Judiciary Committee Immigration Subcommittee. Retrieved August 12, 2002, from *http://leahy.senate.gov/press/200105/010522.html.*

Martin, L., et al. (2001). Who will care for each of us? *Report by Panel on the Future of Health Care Labor in a Graying Society.* Chicago: University of Illinois.

Minnick, A. (2000). Retirement, the nursing workforce and the year 2005. *Nursing Outlook, 48,* 211–217.

Nevidjon, B., & Erikson, J. I. (2001). The nursing shortage: Solutions for the short and long term. *Online Journal of Issues in Nursing, 6*(1), 4.

Sloane, M. M. (1999). Aging nursing faculty adds to RN shortage concerns. *Nursing Spectrum, 9*(5), 18–19.

U.S. Department of Health and Human Services. (1988). *Secretary's Commission on Nursing.* Washington, DC: Office of the Secretary, U.S. Department of Health and Human Services.

Vermont Organization of Nurse Leaders. (2000a). *State of nursing in Vermont: Impact on hospitals.* Presentation to the Public Oversight Commission, Montpelier, Vermont, August 2, 2000.

Vermont Organization of Nurse Leaders. (2000b). *The Current State of Nursing in Vermont.* Killington, Vermont: Vermont Organization of Nurse Leaders.

Wunderlich, G., Sloane, F., & Davis, C. (1996). Nursing staff in hospitals and nursing homes. Is it adequate? *Report of the Institute of Medicine.* Washington, DC: National Academy Press.

CHAPTER TWO

Tackling the Nursing Shortage in Rural Missouri: Linking Education and Service in a Differentiated Practice Environment

Susan W. Devaney, Alice F. Kuehn, Ruth J. Jones, and Lynne Ott

Missouri is among many states experiencing the current nursing shortage crisis, particularly in the rural areas of the state. The population of Missouri in 2000 was 5,595,211, with 1,800,410, or 32% of the total population, living in rural areas (University of Missouri, 2002; U.S. Department of Agriculture, 2002). This reflects a 9% increase in total population from 1990 to 2000, but a 10% increase in rural population during the same time frame; 75% of the registered nurses in Missouri are in the metropolitan areas, compared to 82% nationally (U.S. Department of Health and Human Services, 2000).

Concurrently, hospitals in Missouri have been closing steadily, declining from 150 in 1983 to 124 in 1999. Many of these closings are in rural areas, and the decline is a result of consolidation, small patient volume, and proximity to another facility (Mosley, 1999). Those remaining are struggling to provide care in a time of declining reimbursement and increasing shortage of health care personnel, particularly nurses. In 2001, the registered nurse (RN) vacancy rate in Missouri was 10.8% in the metropolitan areas and 12% in the rural areas. The corresponding licensed practical nurse (LPN) vacancy rate was 11.5% and 8%. The lower LPN vacancy rate in the rural areas may be due to the larger number of practical nursing programs in those areas.

This grim picture of a declining number of nurses is accompanied by the failure of the profession to recruit and retain adequate numbers of new and younger nurses. Actualities of job stress, long hours, staff shortages, and poor working environments are forcing nurses to leave health care facilities. As their stories filter through the media, young people—who often value time over money and loyalty to the work rather than the employer—are choosing other careers (Nevidjon & Erickson, 2001). Add to this mixture: a work arena that perpetuates the motto "A nurse is a nurse is a nurse" with little or no recognition of educational or experiential differences; nurse administrators who lack the leadership, knowledge of change theory, and patience to make changes; and nurse educators who may not understand the complexities of the work setting yet are attempting to prepare credible graduates, and the problem seems insurmountable. The need for new partnerships, new ways of thinking about management, and innovative curricula are needed to keep pace with the immediate and future demands of the health care system (American Association of Colleges of Nursing [AACN], 1993).

BACKGROUND

Fitzgibbon Hospital, a 60-bed acute-care facility located in rural Marshall, Missouri, was facing difficult times by 1996. Like other rural hospitals, it was in danger of closing due to financial and staffing issues. Faced with a 10% budget cut and a 61% nursing turnover rate, the hospital made a decision to introduce shared governance. This collaborative management style includes "balancing power equally between management and staff on the issues related to the professional practice of nursing" (Porter-O'Grady, 1992). A direct result of this action was the formation of the Medical-Surgical Nursing Management Council to assume staffing and scheduling responsibilities. The goal was to work toward implementation of the differentiated practice model described by Koerner and Karpiuk (1994).

Differentiated practice is a concept that acknowledges the practice of professional nursing as having many roles and responsibilities. It also recognizes that nurses have varied educational preparation, expertise and competencies that they bring to the patient care environment. To utilize best the unique contributions of all nursing personnel, differentiated practice creates systems that:

• focus on structuring roles and functions of nurses according to education, experience and competence;

• seek to have the work of nursing carried out by the most appropriate nurse in the most appropriate manner;

• integrate services to provide comprehensive, cost-effective care; and

• stress the key points of accountability, autonomy, nurse role, and shared governance.

In 1997, Fitzgibbon Hospital took the leap by initiating differentiated practice on its medical-surgical unit. The goal was to rebuild the staff and utilize registered nurses in roles that were appropriate for their educational preparation and experience. By 2002, the nursing turnover rate had dropped to 12% for the first two quarters. As the hospital moved forward on the course of implementing this model, nursing workforce development and analysis was the subject of a 6-year, two-phase project at the University of Missouri Sinclair School of Nursing, funded as a Colleagues in Caring site through the Robert Wood Johnson Foundation (http://www.nursingfutures.org). Phase two, which focused on furthering the collaboration between education and service, brought together the staff from Fitzgibbon Hospital and the nursing faculties of the University of Missouri-Columbia Sinclair School of Nursing and Moberly Area Community College.

THE PROJECT

As the work of the Colleagues in Caring project evolved, the two faculty groups began to discuss the development and implementation of a differentiated practice model of education. If students were thrust into environments of differentiation and nursing teams, why not introduce the concept during the educational process? The result was a project funded by the Department of Education Fund for Improvement of Post Secondary Education (FIPSE) and titled University and Community College Partnership. The grant funded curriculum development, and students from both schools began to work together in clinical settings to clarify roles and learn teamwork.

One clinical site selected for the shared experience was Fitzgibbon Hospital. Working with faculty from both programs, hospital administration and staff developed a shared learning experience to reflect the distinctive competency outcomes of the two educational programs. Working in groups of four (two second-year AD students and two seventh-semester BS students), the students participated in a 2-day

TABLE 2.1 Fitzgibbon Hospital Experience Agenda.

Day 1	
7:00–7:30	Welcome and Overview of Fitzgibbon Hospital Nursing Practice Model Lynne Ott, MSN, RN, Vice President of Patient Care Services
7:30–9:45	Students with: Patient Care Coordinator and Utilization Review Coordinator
9:45–10:30	Discharge Planning Meeting with Care Team
10:30–12:00	Students with: Clinical Care Coordinator and Associate Nurse
12:00–1:00	Lunch
1:00–2:30	Students with: Clinical Care Coordinator and Associate Nurse
2:30–3:00	Student/Faculty Conference
Evening Jam Session—Nursing Issues facilitated by Lynne Ott	

Day 2	
6:45–7:15	Supervisory Report—Clinical Care Coordinators
7:15–10:00	Students with: Patient Care Coordinator and Utilization Review Coordinator
10:00–10:30	Discharge Planning Meeting with Care Team
10:30–11:30	Nurse Manager Role
11:30–12:00	Nursing Report Card
12:00–1:00	Lunch
1:00–2:30	Nursing Coordinating Council Meeting
2:30–3:00	Student/Faculty Exit Conference

immersion experience, interacting with nursing staff at all levels in management and clinical positions. The schedule is structured so that students can experience as many of the unique characteristics of the differentiated practice model as possible (see Table 2.1).

On the evening prior to the experience, students received an orientation to the hospital's model. Discussion also centered on the curriculum similarities and differences of the two schools, the history of AD and BS education, the role of the state board, and the purpose of the NCLEX-RN. The faculty member who holds a joint appointment with both participating educational institutions conducted the sessions and supervised students during the experience.

For the next 2 days, students had the opportunity to talk with staff about the differentiated practice model, their work, and the communication patterns necessary for the model to work efficiently. They participated in the shared governance council, discharge planning meetings, and care-plan conferences. An evening "jam session" allowed for discussion with hospital staff about the model and other issues of concern to the students. A student enrolled in the master of science in nursing program at the University of Missouri also joined the group for the session. Questions developed by the faculty and hospital staff included the following: What are your biggest concerns about nursing and your going to work as a nurse? Why did you choose nursing? What do you hope to accomplish as a nurse and how do you plan to do this? What are the major health issues facing our nation and the world? Why do nurses eat their young? What are the pros and cons of utilizing the differentiated practice model? How do we promote teamwork among nurses of various educational levels?

EVALUATION

Following the 2-day session, students completed an evaluation form where they were asked to describe what they learned in response to a set of questions, for example: Did this change my view of nursing? Did it raise new questions to me about my education and the profession? What was my overall impression of the experience? Students were also asked to comment on accommodations, food, and evening activities, and to make suggestions for future groups of students. In addition, a brief focus group session was conducted just prior to departure, affording students an opportunity to make any final comments.

COMMENTS

General comments, including those related to the experience of working with students from another school, the Fitzgibbon staff, and the clinical instructor, have been refreshing and reflect increased knowledge of hospital management. A sample of these comments is as follows:

- I was unsure what to expect from this experience, thinking the role of the AD nurse was seriously downplayed; however, I was excited to see that associate nurses (which includes MSN, BSN, and AD nurses) were appreciated for their contribution to the health care team and were treated with a great deal of respect.
- I learned that each aspect of nursing is trained to perform as a part of the team (as noted by our varying education), and that each team member has strengths that allow for better patient care.
- I have learned more about the leadership and management roles of nursing this past week than in the last 4 years of school.
- I learned what a positive influence and impact nurses can have on the organizational structure and function of a hospital.

- The most important thing I feel I learned is the fact that nurses are more than capable of not only providing patient care, but also running a hospital and making administrative decisions.
- Observing nursing from this structural perspective really made me view the profession from a different angle. Never before had I put so much thought into the organization of nursing. Typically, my focus has been more on actual patient care, rather than the components of the work model. I think this was a very valuable experience for me as I prepare for a future as a professional nurse. It is important for me to begin "thinking" like a nurse.
- One of the most peculiar things my peers and I noticed from the beginning was how happy all of the staff appeared to be. I was amazed at the relative comfort all members of the health care team felt in spite of a very busy workload and several staffing difficulties that had to be overcome.

EMPLOYMENT RESULTS

As a result of this project, three students interviewed for positions at the hospital and began work in summer 2002. In 2003, all were still employed there. At the beginning of the winter 2002 term, the hospital had two RN vacancies. This represented 3.5% of the total RN FTE (total nursing FTE is 99 with 56 of those being RN positions). By the end of the semester, there were no RN vacancies.

DISCUSSION

The most positive result of this project to date has been the opportunity for students to experience a nursing management model that is proactive and whose success is based on teamwork. Additionally, this project has allowed the hospital to showcase the differentiated practice model to future nurses through a unique clinical experience that focuses on management rather than on direct patient care. In a rural area where word-of-mouth often determines where nurses seek employment, the positive experiences of these new graduates have the potential to be very beneficial.

Implementation of this type of management clinical experience requires a shift in faculty thinking to be more focused on management skills. Although many schools have implemented extensive preceptor programs during the final semester in which the student cares for groups of patients, they often focus on personal responsibility for their "team of patients" rather than having a "team of nurses" approach to patient care. Providing opportunities for students to learn caregiving as well as management skills can enhance their contributions as members of the health care team.

There was some initial resistance when faculty in rural Missouri were afforded the opportunity for students to participate in this differentiated practice project in lieu of regularly scheduled clinical practice. For example, there were comments by faculty about students all needing to complete the same clinical experience, and concerns about releasing students from regularly scheduled patient care clinical times. To participate in the project students were at the time enrolled in medical-surgical nursing, pediatrics, and mental health nursing. To accommodate the concerns raised by the faculty, students were offered clinical time in these particular specialty areas in Fitzgibbon Hospital, and were required to submit a written clinical report to the instructor.

A key consideration for success in this type of endeavor is support by the hospital staff. Recognition by staff that this type of experience prior to graduation can reduce anxiety about the first work position and prepare successful graduates is paramount. Further, it is important that all members of the health care team, including physicians, are aware of the project and can answer student questions accurately and appropriately. Students were quick to note the lack of communication and support of some staff. Those who were aware of the student experience willingly talked about their roles and the pros and cons of differentiated practice. A few commented that sharing this information with students reinforced their own excitement about their roles in the evolution of this nursing management model.

Cost is a potentially major issue that must be considered in implementing a differentiated practice model. The low faculty-student ratio (1:6) afforded by this grant-funded pilot project is not likely to be cost-effective for schools of nursing. Faculty and hospital staffs need to think creatively about ways to partner in order to offer students this type of experience, considering both cost and the unique characteristics of the institution. In this project, for example, staff were not required to supervise students directly in patient care roles, and were better able to accommodate the students into their schedules. Cost of this project for the winter semester 2002, excluding faculty salaries, was $1,157 (see Table 2.2).

TABLE 2.2 Cost of Fitzgibbon Hospital Experience.

Food* and Supplies	$79
Mileage	$106
Motel for 16 people	$971
Total cost for 16 people	$1157

*Additional food supplied "in kind" by the hospital

CONCLUSION

By linking an associate degree program and a baccalaureate program through a common clinical experience, this project sought to provide students with a view of a differentiated practice model of nursing. Participation in the project has expanded their view of teamwork and the nursing role. Ideally, this will ease their transition to becoming employees in the clinical practice setting.

The impact on faculty and the nursing programs overall has been subtler. Some changes have been made in the curriculum of both programs. For example, faculties have expressed an increased awareness of the nurse's role and the need to emphasize teamwork in course content. Course revisions have been easier to achieve in the associate degree program, primarily because of the smaller numbers of courses and faculty.

Post-project discussions have ensued regarding ways to continue the project when the grant funding is no longer available. This project and others articulated in the grant have slowly become a part of curriculum reform as students report their experiences to classmates and discussion filters down to those students who have yet to enter senior level coursework. As with other changes in the curriculum, the responsibility of faculty is to keep abreast of the health care system and respond accordingly.

FUTURE PLANS

The experience of learning in a differentiated practice environment continued in the academic year 2002–2003, with the plan to incorporate LPN and MS program students into the project, in both the acute care setting and in two community-based settings. As data are collated and analyzed, it is expected that the project will serve as a model for expansion to school/hospital partners in other geographic locations.

REFERENCES

American Association of Colleges of Nursing. (1993). *Education and practice collaboration: Mandate for quality education, practice and research for health care reform.*

Koerner, J. G., & Karpiuk, K. L. (1994). *Implementing differentiated nursing practice: Transformation by design.* Gaithersburg, MD: Aspen.

Mosley, M. (1999). Patterns in Missouri hospital closings. *Missouri Epidemiologist, 21*(5).

Nevidjon, B., & Erickson, J. (January 31, 2001). The nursing shortage: Solutions for the short and long term. *Online Journal of Issues in Nursing, 6*(1), Manuscript 4. Available: *http://www.nursingworld.org/ojin/topic14/tpc14_4.htm.*

Porter-O'Grady, T. (1992). *Implementing shared governance.* St. Louis, MO: Mosby Year Book.

University of Missouri. Office of Social and Economic Data Analysis. Retrieved April 18, 2002 from the University of Missouri Web site: http://www.oseda.missouri.edu/.

U.S. Department of Agriculture. Economic Research Service. Retrieved April 18, 2002 from *http://www.ers.usda.gov/StateFacts/MO.htm*

U.S. Department of Health and Human Services. (2000). *The registered nurse population* (DHHS Publication No. BHP00168). Washington, DC: U.S. Government Printing Office.

CHAPTER THREE

A Rural State's Response to the Nursing Shortage: Nevada's Story

Julie E. Johnson, Nancy Polatty and Doreen Begley

A lthough Nevada has the fastest growing population in the United States, it also has the dubious distinction of having the worst nursing shortage in the nation. This shortage is exacerbated by several factors. Nevada's population more than doubled from 1990–1999. The Hispanic population has been the fastest growing ethnic group, and much of the population increase consists of retirees and other "golden agers," resulting in a need for more registered nurses. As with the rest of the nation, health care delivery is changing in Nevada with an increase in managed care, a shift from inpatient to outpatient care, and an increase in technology, creating a need to shift the focus of nursing education. State legislative and regulatory efforts to address health care problems, such as the large number of uninsured and underinsured in Nevada, the rise in prescription drug costs, and inpatient staffing concerns increase the need for registered nurses. Finally, although Nevada is unique in having more applicants than available positions for its nursing schools, a shortage in faculty makes it impossible to admit all qualified applicants (Packham, 2001).

The nursing leadership of Nevada has responded to this crisis on several fronts. With the help of the Nevada Hospital Association, legislative efforts, recruitment efforts, increased retainment efforts, and statewide cooperative educational efforts have been initiated. This chapter describes how these efforts came about in the context of Nevada's uniqueness, its system of higher education in general, and nursing education in specific. Although many of these efforts occurred within the context of Nevada's unique situation, we believe that they can be applied in other states that are experiencing a critical nursing shortage.

TRANSFORMATIONAL NURSING LEADERSHIP THEORY

Transformational leadership theory distinguishes between transactional and transformational leadership. Transactional leaders act in response to specific situations, exchanging favors at the leader's bidding to reach the leader's goals. Transformational leaders use the process of change to develop in stakeholders the values and beliefs that support change. This requires that four factors operate in tandem: leaders must know what their own values and beliefs are, they must model these values and beliefs, they must know what must change, and they must understand organizational strengths and ethics. They work to change the organization to be responsive to its needs and those of the public (Kent, Johnson, & Graber, 1998).

Effective transformational leaders have a clear vision of where the organization is going, how it needs to change, and what is needed to effect those changes. They communicate their vision by their words and their actions, changing the way people think about their lives and their work. They encourage creative ideas and improvement of all facets of the organization. Transformational leaders also establish partnerships and work with groups outside the organization to implement change. These leaders take the long view and work to promote maximum buy-in of such changes by internal stakeholders (e.g., health care organizations, nursing students and faculty, professional organization leaders and members, and administrative leaders) and external stakeholders (e.g., patients, taxpayers, political groups and office holders, and the general public). They build confidence and increase energy within the organization through their positive spirit, persistence, and perseverance. Finally, transformational leaders are able to maintain their focus on the desired outcome (Kent et al., 1998).

Nursing leaders in Nevada, including the directors of the schools of nursing, nursing leaders in health care organizations and professional associations, and administrative leaders, such as the Nevada Board of Nursing and the Nevada Hospital Association, have been working within the existing organization—the nursing system—to respond to the nursing shortage crisis. As demonstrated below, they are transformational leaders seeking to change both the organization and the values and beliefs of its stakeholders.

THE STATE OF NEVADA

Nevada's 17 counties comprise an area of 110,540 square miles, making it the seventh largest state in the nation. Of these 17 counties, 10 are classified as frontier with population densities averaging 1.46 persons per square mile, four are designated as rural, and three are urban. The cities of Reno and Las Vegas, approximately 485 miles apart, are Nevada's largest urban areas. Eighty-seven percent of Nevada's land is federally controlled, making it unavailable for development or taxation; thus revenues to support higher education must be garnered from other sources.

Coupled with its unique geographic features, Nevada is projected to remain the fastest growing state in the nation for the next 25 years (Nevada State Demographer's Office, 2000). Clark County, where Las Vegas is located, is one of the fastest growing counties in the nation. Nevada also has the fastest growing population of older adults, who tend to be the greatest consumers of health care services.

HIGHER EDUCATION IN NEVADA

One coordinated and collaborative organization, the University and Community College System of Nevada (UCCSN), provides higher education in Nevada. The UCCSN contains two universities, four community colleges, and one 4-year college. The University of Nevada, Reno, located in northern Nevada, is the land-grant institution for the state. Other institutions in the UCCSN are the University of Nevada, Las Vegas (485 miles southeast of Reno), Truckee Meadows Community College in Reno; Western Nevada Community College in Carson City (30 miles south of Reno), Great Basin College in Elko (290 miles east of Reno), and the Community College of Southern Nevada in Las Vegas. Nevada State College, Henderson (several miles from Las Vegas) opened in fall 2002. Currently, six of the seven institutions offer nursing programs. Nevada State College plans to implement its program in fall 2003, bringing the number of nursing schools in the state to seven.

In 2002, the combined enrollment in the state's six nursing programs was 762. The majority of students are Nevada residents and reflect the ethnic composition of the state: 84.8% White, 6.5% Asian or Pacific Islander, 6.0% Hispanic, 2.5% African American, and 0.2% Native American.

NEVADA'S NURSING SHORTAGE

Although there are 782 registered nurses per 100,00 population nationally, Nevada has only 580, the fewest in the nation (Nevada Hospital Association, 2000). There are several causes for the state's critical nursing shortage.

First, Nevada's population is growing faster than nursing programs in the UCCSN are currently able to produce new graduates. According to the Nevada Hospital Association (Packham, 2001), 662 nurses per year are needed for the period 2000 to 2008 to accommodate the projected increase in population and attrition of nurses who are currently employed. Yet, only about 262 students graduate from Nevada schools of nursing annually. The low number of graduates is attributed to several factors. First, the Nevada State Board of Nursing mandates a faculty/student ratio of 1:8 in the clinical setting. Thus, enrollments must be limited unless schools are able to hire more faculty to teach in the practice setting. To date, additional state funded lines given to the UCCSN have not been allocated to nursing.

Second, the nationwide faculty shortage and low salaries compared to those in the practice setting have made it difficult for some schools in the system to recruit more faculty. Third, new hospital construction has contributed to the projected nursing shortage in Nevada. Within the next 3 years, five new hospitals with a combined bed capacity of 676 will open in the Las Vegas area in order to meet the health care needs of its increasing population. This increased bed capacity was not known when it was predicted that Nevada would need an additional 662 nurses per year for 2000 to 2008.

Last, the aging nursing workforce exacerbates the nursing shortage (Buerhaus, Staiger, & Auerbach, 2000). More than 50% of Nevada's nurses are over the age of 46, and fewer than 10% are under 25 (Nevada State Board of Nursing, 1999). Thus, the state's largest cohort of nurses is entering its retirement years without a significant number of new graduates to replace it.

NEVADA RESPONDS TO THE SHORTAGE

In 1999, the Nevada Hospital Association; founded a statewide task force to address the nursing shortage. Membership includes the executive director of the Nevada Hospital Association; the nurse executive of the Nevada Hospital Association, a representative of the state's two university schools of nursing; a representative of the state's four community college nursing programs; a regent from the UCCSN; a state legislator and three aides to U.S. Senators, the executive director of the Nevada State Board of Nursing; the president of the Nevada Nurses Association; the executive director of the Western Interstate Commission on Higher Education; and the health policy analyst for the

Nevada State Office of Rural Health. Representatives of Nevada's hospital chief executive officers and chief nursing officers represent the state's rural hospitals, large medical centers, and smaller hospitals. Using transformational leadership theory, this task force recognized that any solution to the nursing shortage must involve cooperation, collaboration, and trust among all nursing organizations, for example, schools of nursing, hospitals, nursing associations, and regulatory agencies. They also recognized that its members had to model this cooperation, collaboration, and trust to implement the organizational and belief changes needed to adequately respond to the nursing shortage (Kent et al., 1998).

During its first 2 years, the task force met every month for about 4 hours. Meetings alternated between Reno and Las Vegas. Initially, the task force charged one of its members with determining the current and projected status of the nursing workforce and nursing education in the state. Data were collected from a variety of sources, including the Nevada State Board of Nursing, Nevada Department of Education and Training, and schools of nursing in the UCCSN. Based on the findings, the task force made numerous recommendations regarding the educational system, employers of nurses, state government agencies, and professional associations in Nevada. Findings and recommendations were included in a written report entitled *The Nursing Workforce and Education in Nevada* (Packham, 2001).

Recognizing that implementing the needed changes would create an opportunity to engage both internal and external stakeholders to commit to the change (Kent et al., 1998), the task force organized two forums, one in Reno in March 2001 and one in Las Vegas in June 2001. These forums were well attended by nurses, nursing faculty, and nursing students, and invited representatives from K–12 programs, UCCSN, employers of nurses, regulators, legislators, and the media. The task force presented their study findings (Packham, 2001), and attendees developed and discussed the following recommendations:

• Expand and or reallocate financial resources for all UCCSN nursing schools.
• Increase funding for nursing faculty, program needs, equipment, scholarships, and loan repayments.
• Increase efforts to recruit and retain minority and other nontraditional students into nursing.
• Improve articulation agreements among Nevada's schools of nursing and high schools and community colleges.
• Provide state-funded summer salaries for UCCSN nursing faculty.
• Provide clinical placements and preceptors commensurate with the expansion of the UCCSN nursing education programs.

• Promote career ladders and financial support for non-RN health care personnel to transition into UCCSN nursing programs.

• Recruit graduate students into the nursing education options at the two universities to alleviate the faculty shortage in community colleges.

• Review state regulations impacting nursing education and practice.

• Provide a supportive work environment to encourage nurses to remain in the profession.

• Heighten the public's awareness of Nevada's nursing shortage and its implications for health care.

• Develop strategies to improve the public's image of the nursing profession.

The forums had two significant outcomes. First, to act on the above recommendations, the task force established several subcommittees: (a) Professional Development, to address educational issues; (b) Attraction, to address recruitment; and (c) Commitment, to address retention. Membership on the subcommittees was open to nurses and students throughout the state. Task force members from Reno and Las Vegas cochair these subcommittees, which meet monthly via videoconference. Nursing educators, nursing administrators, staff nurses, nursing students, and community members have become active on all three subcommittees. This process created an involved group of stakeholders who have a definite interest and investment in the organization and the process. As seen below, these committee members have demonstrated their commitment to the process by giving their time and energy and using creative problem-solving skills to develop useful and workable strategies (Kent, Johnson & Graber, 1998).

Second, by establishing working partnerships and relationships with both federal and state officeholders, Assembly Bill 378, which directed UCCSN to develop a plan to double enrollments in entry level nursing programs by 2006, was passed by the 2001 legislature. Though it was not funded, several legislators were active sponsors of Assembly Bill 378, and have committed themselves to efforts to fund this mandate. These partnerships and relationships created an involved group of external stakeholders who are invested in the success of the process (Kent, Johnson & Graber, 1998).

Through these outcomes, progress is being made in addressing Nevada's nursing shortage. For example, in the past year the Professional Development Subcommittee reviewed the articulation agreements between the universities and community colleges. To facilitate transfers between schools of nursing, the directors have explored ways to ensure that as many prerequisite courses as possible are in common across the campuses. The subcommittee also worked with the Nevada Board of Nursing to enable graduate students enrolled in a nursing education option to obtain clinical teaching experience in associate degree programs.

In fall 2002, Nevada State College opened in Henderson. The director of its school of nursing has adopted the upper-division curriculum offered at the University of Nevada, Reno. Students will be able to transfer between the two institutions without delaying their graduation. The first nursing class will be admitted in fall 2003.

Professional Development Subcommittee members also negotiated with the State Board of Nursing to reexamine mandated faculty/student ratios in precepted clinical settings. An agreement was reached whereby annually the directors can request that the ratio be increased in leadership and community health experiences. This flexibility allows a more efficient use of faculty as enrollments increase without jeopardizing public safety.

The Attraction Subcommittee is conducting a campaign to recruit potential students into nursing. They are using age appropriate coloring books in elementary schools and videos and brochures in middle and high schools. In summer 2002, the subcommittee expanded the nurse camps, and more than 700 high school students attended to explore nursing as a profession. Despite this, the Attraction Subcommittee is moving slowly because student recruitment is not a major concern in Nevada. Currently, the University of Nevada, Las Vegas has approximately 700 declared prenursing majors; the University of Nevada, Reno has about 500; and Truckee Meadows Community College has approximately 600.

Because Nevada's nursing shortage has had the greatest impact on acute care facilities, the Commitment Subcommittee has made recommendations regarding staff retention to be used by hospitals throughout the state. Their primary thrust is to create a safe environment for open discussion between nurses and administrators. The subcommittee also created the Chief Retention Officer Pilot Program to develop ways to retain staff currently employed by the institution. About 20 hospitals statewide are participating in the program. If these strategies are successful, they can be used by other health care agencies, such as nursing homes and public health departments.

The second major outcome, the passage of AB378, prompted the Chancellor of the UCCSN to request that the director of the University of Nevada, Reno Orvis School of Nursing and the nurse executive of the Nevada Hospital Association develop the plan to double nursing enrollments in the UCCSN. Working collaboratively with Nevada's seven schools of nursing and the UCCSN Board of Regents Health Care Education Committee, and with the support of the chancellor's office and the Nevada Hospital Association, the plan was developed over a 6-month period. The Board of Regents unanimously approved the plan in August 2002, and it is part of their 2003 budget request to the legislature. At the time of this writing, the plan was in the governor's office awaiting the start of the January 2003 session.

The goal of the plan is to double the number of students enrolled in the UCCSN schools of nursing by 2006–2007. Because the majority of schools in the UCCSN have had to deny admission to qualified applicants due to lack of program capacity over the past several years, increasing enrollments is not expected to be a problem. Indeed, the number of students enrolled in prenursing courses suggests that several schools could double their enrollments immediately if funding was available to hire faculty.

To double the enrollments, the plan requests $12 million in 2003–2005 and $14 million in 2005–2007, for a total of $26 million. Not surprisingly, the majority of the funding will be used to hire additional faculty and staff, renovate buildings as needed to accommodate growth, and purchase additional equipment and supplies.

Two components of the plan are critical to its success. First, tutoring programs in English, mathematics, and science must be developed to assure the success of at-risk and English-as-second-language students who want to enroll in nursing. Second, the summer session must be state funded. At present it is not, which makes it impossible for schools of nursing in Nevada to offer summer courses. As a result, clinical sites are filled to capacity during the fall and spring semesters and are not used at all during the summer session. These sites are unable to accommodate doubled enrollments during the traditional school year without the use of creative scheduling. Working through the task force, all clinical agencies supported and cooperated in efforts to place students in facilities using 12-hour shifts, weekends, and nights throughout the year. Schools are also planning to admit students two to three times a year, offer accelerated programs, and provide remedial instruction in written and verbal communication for English-as-second-language students when the summer session is fully state funded.

In addition to the critical needs for tutoring and summer funding, the plan proposes creative strategies that are common to all Nevada schools of nursing, as well as those that are unique to each school. This modeling of cooperation and collaboration is an essential part of transformational leadership. The nursing leaders of Nevada have communicated their vision through their actions, and have created a positive atmosphere by modeling confidence and will (Kent et al., 1998). Common strategies include:

- an aggressive statewide media campaign, coordinated by the UCCSN Chancellor's office, to recruit students into nursing;
- collaboration with school districts throughout the state to identify potential nursing students and assign them nurse mentors to encourage them to pursue their interest in nursing;
- collaboration with school districts to offer certain courses, such as medical terminology, for concurrent high school and college credit;
- the use of distance education modalities and innovative alternative class scheduling to teach prerequisite courses; and
- collaboration with the Western Interstate Commission on Higher Education to assist students to obtain a doctorate and then to return to the faculty.

Strategies that are unique to one or more of the campuses in the UCCSN include faculty sharing between several schools of nursing and the development of a cooperative online doctoral program in nursing with other interested universities in the western United States. One school proposes to offer its program on weekends during the fall and spring semesters, while another will offer its program during the evening hours. Two community colleges and one university are planning to make dual patient assignments between associate and baccalaureate students to capitalize on the strengths of each program, to allow students to provide care from their program's unique perspectives, and to utilize faculty better.

The statewide task force, its subcommittees, and Nevada's schools of nursing are implementing programs to address the nursing shortage during the time that the plan to double enrollments proceeds through the legislative process. In 2001, the University of Nevada, Reno Orvis School of Nursing received funding from the Nevada Hospital Association to admit eight additional qualified students to its new accelerated bachelor's program for second degree students. In 2002, Reno Orvis received funding from Nevada Works, a federal workforce development agency, to hire three faculty and admit 24 students to the accelerated program. The grant is also intended to demonstrate to the state legislature that, with funding, Nevada's schools of nursing are able to admit qualified students who would otherwise have to delay their entry into the program or leave the state to receive their education.

In January 2002, the school added an education option to its graduate program so that community colleges will have larger pools from which to recruit faculty. Students receive part of their teaching practicum under the guidance of community college faculty. There is similar activity in the southern part of the state. For example, the University of Nevada, Las Vegas Department of Nursing is collaborating with the Clark County School District, the Community College of Southern Nevada, and a large medical center to offer a mentoring program for elementary- and high-school students who are interested nursing. The department also receives funding from a medical center in Las Vegas to employ faculty holding joint appointments, and is planning to reopen its education option in the graduate program.

EVALUATION

Evaluation of these organizational changes is ongoing. The first measure of success will be the extent to which the plan to double enrollments in UCCSN schools of nursing is funded by the 2003 legislature. The second measure will be the continued implementation of the common and unique strategies by UCCSN schools of nursing, as described above. Achievements of the Professional Development, Attraction, and Commitment subcommittees of the Nursing Institute of Nevada are monitored on a continuing basis.

CONCLUSION

Nevada's severe nursing shortage has galvanized those in the state who have a deep concern for the health of its citizens. Organizations that in the past have been at odds with one another or have felt the need to compete have put aside their differences. They have made a strong commitment to work collaboratively to address the shortage and meet the state's needs for nursing care.

Nevada's nursing leaders have become transformational leaders to meet the nursing shortage crisis. They have created a vision of what must happen to solve this crisis, communicated this vision through their words and actions, and developed creative actions to solve the crisis through task force subcommittees and through other common and unique strategies. Students, faculty, and administrators of Nevada's schools of nursing, health care organizations, professional organization leaders and members, and administrative leaders as internal stakeholders are involved in, and are committed to, the vision and actions. External stakeholders—the citizens of Nevada and their elected representatives—are becoming more and more aware of the implications of the nursing shortage, and will need to commit the resources needed to resolve the crisis. The leaders are working to build confidence and energy within the organization by encouraging and modeling positive spirit and will. They are maintaining their focus on the critical need in Nevada to increase the number of qualified and competent nurses (Kent et al., 1998).

In 2002, the statewide task force incorporated and became the Nursing Institute of Nevada, making it eligible for a variety of funding opportunities. The institute will also be a key player in convincing the legislature to fund the plan to double nursing school enrollments. Members of the Nursing Institute are convinced that Nevada's nursing crisis

> demands a major and sustained financial response from state policy makers and the University and Community College System of Nevada. It must be stressed that dealing with this shortage will not come cheap or quickly. Nonetheless, the price of inaction will ultimately be born by all Nevadans at some point in time. (Packham, 2002)

They are determined that Nevadans will not pay the price with their health.

REFERENCES

Buerhaus, P. I., Staiger, D. O., & Auerbach, D. I. (2000). Implications of an aging registered nurse workforce. *Journal of the American Medical Association, 283,* 2948–2954.

Kent, T., Johnson, J. A., & Graber, D.R. (1998). Leadership in the formation of new health care environments. In E. C. Hein, (Ed.), *Contemporary leadership behavior: Selected readings* (5th ed.). Philadelphia: Lippincott. Nevada Hospital Association (2000). NHA survey on efforts in nursing. Reno, NV: Author.

Nevada State Board of Nursing (1999). *Nevada State Board of Nursing annual report 98–99.* Reno, NV: Author.

Nevada State Demographer's Office (2000). *Nevada county population projections 2000 to 2010.* Reno, NV: Author.

Packham, J. F. (2001). The nursing workforce and nursing education in Nevada. Reno, NV: Nevada Hospital Association.

Packham, J. F. (2002, February 19). Deal with the health care crisis now or pay later. *Reno Gazette-Journal,* pp. 5.1–5.16.

CHAPTER FOUR

The Shortage of Operating Room Nurses: What AORN Is Doing About It

Suzanne C. Beyea

T he presence of the registered professional nurse in the operating room (OR) promotes the health and safety of surgical patients. The Association of periOperative Registered Nurses (AORN) has grave concerns about the worsening shortage of qualified health care perioperative personnel, specifically professional nurses (American Hospital Association [AHA], 2001). AORN members have voiced concerns about and provided anecdotal reports of patient injuries, or "near-misses," related to staffing shortages. Increasing numbers of reports are received about delays or the cancellation of surgery due to inadequate staffing. AORN members are also concerned about the increased burden placed on OR nurses to work extra hours, take more call hours, or work in unsafe conditions. In response to these issues, the AORN board of directors has committed organizational resources to provide member support and develop resources to assist members address local, regional, and national shortages of nurses, specifically OR nurses.

The current nursing shortage is the result of a confluence of at least three major factors:

- declining nursing school enrollments
- an aging workforce
- competition for skilled personnel

Note: Adapted with permission. *AORN Journal* 76 (August 2002) © AORN, Inc, Denver, CO.

It is expected that during the next two decades, the nursing shortage will increase because many RNs will enter their 50s and 60s and eventually retire. This overall shortage has contributed significantly to shortages of personnel in the OR (Kimball & O'Neil, 2001).

According to a recent analysis of 16 major studies examining the nursing shortage, the shortage is real, past solutions are inadequate, and a workforce and public health crisis loom in the future. These analyses also indicate that the nursing shortage is present throughout the United States, with the exception of Montana (Kimball & O'Neil, 2001). Factors causing the current and worsening shortage in the OR include

- an aging workforce with many current and imminent retirements;
- a lack of surgical educational content and clinical experiences for nursing students;
- demands for professional nurses in ambulatory care surgical settings; and
- difficulty attracting and keeping perioperative nurses.
  (Buerhaus, Staiger, & Auerbach, 2000)

Although these factors exist in numerous clinical areas, their effects seems more dramatic in the OR and other specialty nursing areas, such as the emergency room and critical care. Many anecdotal and quantitative reports provide evidence of this shortage in perioperative settings with RN vacancy rates reported up to 35%. For example, when 1,500 VHA perioperative leaders were surveyed, 57% of respondents reported vacant RN nursing positions within the ORS in their organizations. The average number of vacancies was five to nine positions and respondents reported that it took on the average of 5 months to fill such a position (Voluntary Hospitals of America [VHA], 2000). Further, a Florida Hospital Association study reports that 82.1% of hospitals report a shortage of operating room nurses (Florida Hospital Association, 2001).

Two studies conducted for Surgical Information Systems (SIS) by the Gallup Organization provide further evidence regarding the nursing shortage in the operating room. In August 1999, SIS reported that OR directors (n = 405) were experiencing an average of 2.1 unfilled full-time nurse positions (Gallup, 1999). Subsequently, in January 2001 SIS reported that OR directors (n = 401) were experiencing an average of 1.4 unfilled full-time nurse positions (Gallup, 2001). These figures suggest that operating rooms are experiencing a shortage of qualified nursing staff. In both studies, OR directors reported the lack of qualified nurses as their biggest concern with regard to the future of OR nursing. Shortages, such as those reported by SIS and VHA, indicate that hospitals may be routinely delaying or postponing elective surgeries because there is an insufficient number of qualified nurses to care for the patient or to staff the OR suite.

CHALLENGE TO PREPARE NEW NURSES FOR THE OR

AORN believes that nurses bring a unique body of knowledge to perioperative settings. Furthermore, the association recognizes that professional RNs contribute significantly to cost-effective, efficient, quality, and safe care in the perioperative setting. The membership of AORN recognizes the need to create pathways and opportunities for students and experienced nurses to learn about OR nursing and to gain the required education and skills.

AORN recognizes the challenge for nursing programs to justify an OR experience in an already tight curricula. The members of the AORN are committed to the premise that the operating room provides a unique opportunity for students to (a) learn surgical asepsis; (b) apply knowledge of anatomy, physiology, and pathophysiology to understand the patient's surgical procedure, its effects on the patient, and the patient's pre- and postoperative needs; (c) recognize the ethical and legal responsibilities of the professional nurse; (d) participate as a member of a multidisciplinary team; (e) learn about the increasing role of technology in the provision of health care; and (f) develop the role of patient advocate. AORN and its members support student experiences such as senior practicum or summer elective or internships in the OR. Faculty members who provide basic students with these types of opportunities have reported that students develop their knowledge and skills in the operating room, ambulatory surgery units, postanesthesia care units, and other perioperative settings.

AORN believes that it plays a critical role in addressing the national nursing shortage and, specifically, the shortage of perioperative RNs by supporting members, educators, and leaders in recruiting new nurses to this specialty. The approach to addressing the nursing shortage must be multidimensional and requires highly collaborative efforts of key stakeholders, including nursing faculty, staff nurses, legislators, and hospital and department administrators. AORN has committed organizational resources to identify and create solutions to address this growing concern and has worked to support members in their efforts to mentor new nurses to the specialty practice in the OR and within related perioperative settings.

AORN'S RESPONSE

During the past 5 years, every department at AORN headquarters has been involved in activities specifically designed to address the nursing shortage. Efforts have been undertaken in various areas, including education, public relations, government affairs and advocacy, membership, and nursing practice and research.

EDUCATION

In 1999, AORN developed and implemented a fully integrated curriculum for nurses who do not have OR experience. This course, Perioperative Nursing Course 101, is presented in a scripted, modular format and consists of 26 educational topics, PowerPoint slides, posttests, and text reading assignments. The course, which uses the "train the trainer" concept, has been implemented in more than 300 clinical settings. More than 1,300 participants have enrolled in the course in hospitals, freestanding ambulatory surgery settings, pediatric specialty hospitals, and academic settings. Contact hours are awarded to participants, and the course is suitable for awarding academic credit. AORN also publishes a core curriculum and produces numerous educational programs on videotape that address the knowledge and clinical skills required by perioperative nurses. These serve as introductory or review resources and can be valuable tools for organizations that choose to design their own educational programs. Additionally, AORN provides a Web-based directory of perioperative nursing courses for students and nurses interested in a career in perioperative nursing. This directory links to the AORN Foundation Web site for scholarship information and to other nursing sites (http://www.aorn.org/foundation/default.htm). In the last calendar year, the AORN Foundation supported scholarships to 39 students pursuing a degree in nursing as well as 74 other registered nurses completing a baccalaureate, master's, or doctoral degree.

AORN also has sponsored numerous workshops and education sessions on recruiting and retaining staff members at its fall conferences and annual congress meeting each spring. Association members actively work with schools of nursing to support perioperative experiences for students and to increase the emphasis on surgical content. For example, members have made contact with a school of nursing and worked to develop collaborative agreements to precept student nurses' clinical experiences. AORN's National Committee on Education is developing a tool kit for members to use when promoting the inclusion of perioperative content in nursing school curricula.

To help AORN members develop mentoring skills, the association has provided numerous education sessions and Journal articles specific to mentoring to assist staff nurses to support students and new staff members. At AORN's 2002 congress, the association offered free registration to student nurses, and approximately 120 students attended. Students were offered a full-day course on understanding the OR. This course was taught by experts in the field and provided hands-on instruction on such topics as gowning and gloving, skin preparation, and electrosurgery.

Also at the 2002 congress, a number of sessions focused on the nursing shortage and recruitment and retention. These sessions included "Peer mentoring for retention"; "Recruitment and retention: Specialty teams and manager emotional intelligence"; and "Today's OR: What works." A number of clinical innovation posters were displayed as well, including "A Clinical Immersion Program in Perioperative Nursing"; "A Key to Success: Building a Perioperative Nurse Consortium"; "Closing the Circle: Caring about Recruiting, Preparing, and Retaining Future Perioperative Nurses"; and "Collaborating to Address a Perioperative Nursing Shortage." In July 2002, AORN's chapter leadership meeting focused on perioperative nursing opportunities, the image of nursing, attracting young nurses, recruitment, retention, morale, multigenerational issues, and mentoring. Attendees at this meeting learned skills that will assist them to recruit and retain nursing staff members and mentor new learners in the OR.

PUBLIC RELATIONS

AORN supports and participates in Nurses for a Healthier Tomorrow, a coalition of nursing and health care organizations. This coalition focuses on creating communication programs targeted to encourage people to consider nursing as a career. The purpose of this project is to communicate the tremendous number of opportunities in nursing as well as present the social importance and career satisfaction that can be found in the nursing profession. The coalition maintains a Web site at http://www.nursesource.org, where further information can be obtained regarding this effort.

AORN promoted Johnson & Johnson's nurse recruitment efforts entitled "The Campaign for Nursing's Future." AORN's executive director, president, and board members attended Johnson and Johnson's stakeholder meeting launching this $20 million multiyear campaign to attract more people to nursing. AORN has alerted its members of the resources and materials provided by Johnson & Johnson and published information about their Web site (http://www.discovernursing.com) and national advertising campaign.

An active public-relations campaign about the nursing shortage, consisting of journal and newsletter articles and news releases, is conducted with AORN members. The association has placed news articles about perioperative nursing in several general newspapers throughout the country. These articles address the role of the registered nurse in the OR, opportunities for OR nurses, educational opportunities to become an OR nurse, and information about AORN's Perioperative 101 course. In addition, both the *AORN Journal* and Surgical Services Management (*SSM*) have published numerous articles regarding the nursing shortage and retention strategies.

Currently, AORN distributes a videotape program for prospective students titled *Nursing: The Ultimate Adventure, Perioperative Edition*. This videotape discusses opportunities in the nursing profession. A career-oriented brochure, *Consider a Career in the OR as a Perioperative Nurse* is also available. AORN has a career packet that provides resources for conducting a job search, interviewing, and writing resumés. The association also sponsors Perioperative Nurse Week each year in November. These activities are designed to encourage perioperative nurses to share information about their specialty with the general public, support health care facilities, and recognize the contributions of perioperative nurses.

GOVERNMENT AFFAIRS AND ADVOCACY

The Government Affairs Department monitors legislation on staffing, funding related to nursing education, and health and safety at both federal and state levels. AORN has joined 45 other nursing organizations in endorsing a consensus statement: "Assuring quality health care for the United States: Supporting nurse education and training, building an adequate supply of nurses." Developed by the Americans for Nursing Shortage Relief (ANSR), an ad hoc group, this statement identifies factors contributing to the nursing crisis and was discussed in the "Health Policy Issues" column of the November 2001 *AORN Journal*. Through its association with other nursing organizations in the ANSR alliance, AORN has continued to support passage of federal legislation and responsible public-policy action to alleviate the nursing shortage, including the Nurse Retention and Quality of Care Act of 2002 (i.e., HR 4654).

In April 2002, ANSR sent a letter to the House and Senate committees that passed HR3487 and S1864, requesting the immediate appointment of the conference committee and passage of the Nurse Reinvestment Act. ANSR supported the Senate version of the bill, including facilitation of the entry of new nurses into the profession, enhancement of the practice environment through implementation of best practices, promotion of faculty development, and improvement of the public image of nursing to encourage its selection as a career.

MEMBERSHIP

AORN has been actively recruiting students to join the association. In June 2001, the board of directors approved a student dues rate of $20 annually. More than 200 students have joined AORN to date as a result. The association maintains an active presence at national and local National Student Nurse Association events. At these events, AORN staffs an exhibit booth and provides information to students about many diverse opportunities in perioperative nursing practice, including the OR, postanesthesia care unit, endoscopy departments, ambulatory surgery units, minimally invasive surgery, and outpatient surgical settings. In addition, AORN leaders and invited speakers present sessions on perioperative topics including the wide range of employment opportunities, robotics in the operating room, and pain control throughout the perioperative experience.

In November 2001, AORN was invited by the American College of Surgeons (ACS) to discuss the nursing shortage. This invitation was a direct result of conversations that AORN's then vice president had with physicians at the ACS annual meeting a month earlier. AORN's then president, vice president, and executive director represented the association at this meeting. Approximately 40 physicians and staff members from 15 surgical specialty groups were present. After introductory remarks from AORN representatives, the group held a wide-ranging discussion about the nursing shortage, its root causes, the impact it is having on the OR, and initiatives to address the shortage. All agreed that the shortage is a serious problem for the OR. Surgeon comments tended to focus on legislative action and reimbursement, and AORN members' comments focused more on work environment issues. Both groups mentioned the importance of education and training at all levels. Patient safety also was a common theme and concern.

NURSING PRACTICE AND RESEARCH

AORN's executive director and staff members from the Center for Nursing Practice and the research department have been involved actively in the Call to the Nursing Profession efforts related to the nursing shortage. AORN was one of more than 60 nursing organizations that participated in a 3-day meeting that was designed to bring the nursing community together to address the shortage. During this meeting, discussions revolved around 10 domains identified as key issues of concern for nurses, the profession, and the public: leadership and planning; delivery systems; legislation, regulation, policy; professional/nursing culture; recruitment and retention; economic value; work environment; public relations and communication; education; and diversity. AORN serves on the steering committee for this national effort and as a co-champion for the activities related to recruitment and retention. The association has contributed work plans to three domains—public relations, public policy, and recruitment and retention—and participates in regular conference calls with representatives from various nursing organizations to implement work plans.

AORN's research department has compiled an extensive reference list related to the nursing shortage as well as research articles related to nurse staffing and patient outcomes. These materials are available to other staff members as well as organizational members. AORN collects reports and articles specific to the nursing shortage in perioperative settings. The department also has collected various state-specific reports and monographs about the nursing shortage with the help of AORN's library staff members. These materials are available in the AORN research department to assist members if they have specific questions about nursing recruitment and retention in their state or region.

Past president Allen and AORN's director of research published an article titled "The Nursing Shortage in the Operating Room and Other Surgical Settings" in the June 2002 issue of the *Bulletin of the American College of Surgeons* (Allen & Beyea, 2002). The article addresses research related to the nursing shortage as well as its etiology and AORN's activities to address this growing crisis. This article was written to describe the status of the nursing shortage and the causative reasons for the crisis in perioperative settings.

CONCLUSION

The nursing shortage in the operating room is real and there are reports of its worsening. AORN members have voiced grave concerns about the growing shortage of qualified nurses. The ever increasing number of adverse events, such as wrong site surgery, has made the need for qualified, experienced nurses even more acute. If the shortage is not addressed, patient safety in the operating room may be further compromised. Clinicians, educators, legislators, and organizational leaders must work collaboratively to develop and implement strategies to address this problem while identifying new initiatives with other professional organizations and industry partners. AORN remains committed to the belief that every perioperative patient deserves a well-qualified, competent RN.

REFERENCES

Allen, S. L., & Beyea, S. C. (2002). The nursing shortage in the operating room and other surgical settings. *Bulletin of the American College of Surgeons, 87,* 8–12.

American Hospital Association. (2001). The hospital workforce: Immediate and future. *AHA Trend Watch, 3*(2), 1–8.

Buerhaus, P., Staiger, D., & Auerbach, D. (2000). Why are shortages of hospital RNs concentrated in specialty care units? *Nursing Economics, 18*(3), 111–116.

Florida Hospital Association. (2001): *Florida's nursing shortage: It is here and it is getting worse.* Florida Hospital Association.

Gallup Organization. (1999). Surgical Information System's operating room directors study. Atlanta, GA: Gallup Poll.

Gallup Organization. (2001). Surgical Information System's operating room directors study: Atlanta, GA: Gallup Poll.

Kimball B., O'Neil, E. (2001). The evolution of a crisis: nursing in America. *Policy. Politics, & Nursing Practice, 2*(3), 180–186.

Voluntary Hospitals of America Inc. (2000). Operating room survey results. Irving, TX: VHA.

PART TWO

The Education Front

CHAPTER FIVE

The Role of Nursing Schools in Addressing the Shortage

Barbara R. Heller and Leslie P. Lichtenberg

T here is a new reality for nursing in the twenty-first century. It is defined by a protracted and complex workforce shortage that is considered to be one of the most damaging health care crises of our time. Dramatic declines in enrollments and graduations are contributing to an unprecedented reduction in the nursing pipeline. Despite recent gains, enrollments at nursing schools nationwide plummeted 17% between 1995 and 2000 (American Association of Colleges of Nursing [AACN], 2002b). Compounding the problem is a growing shortage of nursing school faculty. A recent survey conducted by the Council on Collegiate Education for Nursing (CCEN), Southern Regional Education Board (CCEN, 2001) reported a bleak picture about the supply of nurse educators, highlighting resignations, retirements, and a smaller pool of graduates prepared to teach and recruit at all levels as the primary causes of the faculty shortage.

A myriad of demographic, social, and economic factors have contributed to the nursing crisis, among them an aging population. Life expectancy is at an all-time high, according to a recent report issued by the U.S. Department of Health and Human Services (2002), which cites declines in infant mortality rates and infectious diseases, as well as progress in the management of heart disease, stroke, and injuries as some of the related reasons. Not all older Americans are enjoying good health in their later years, however, and an increase in chronic illnesses and higher acuity levels in hospital-based care can be anticipated as baby boomers age. As these trends continue to emerge, so too will the demand for qualified nurses.

Of course, the graying of America also includes the nursing work-force. Moreover, physical demands, stressful work environments, and long hours are producing job burnout at alarming rates and prevent-ing nurses from working much past their mid-50s. According to Kim-ball and O'Neil, whose recent report *Health Care's Human Crisis: The American Nursing Shortage* (2002) provides an in-depth study of the nursing shortage in 15 markets throughout the country, the nurse population, with an average age of 44, will see many among their ranks retire within the next decade.

Additional contributing factors to the nursing shortage include outdated perceptions about the profession and an abundance of alter-native career opportunities for young women. Moreover, there has been a sea change in health care delivery over the past few years. As a result of an emphasis on managed care, hospital stays are becoming dangerously shorter, shifting the burden of patient care out of hospi-tals and into the community, homes, and ambulatory settings. The American Hospital Association reports that 126,000 nurses are needed to fill vacancies in hospitals nationwide, and there is little relief in sight (American Hospital Association [AHA], 2001). The U.S. Bureau of Labor Statistics projects that more than 1 million new and replace-ment nurses will be needed by the year 2010 (U.S. Bureau of Labor Statistics, 2001).

SEEKING SOLUTIONS

The broad range of issues driving the nursing shortage requires a new approach to producing not only more graduates, but also ones who are better prepared for the challenges of today's changing health care environment. Coffman and colleagues (Coffman, Spetz, Seago, Rose-noff, & O'Neil, 2001) suggest that "nursing schools are an important part of both the problem and the solution" (p. iv) to the nursing shortage. Although efforts to expand student enrollments have already been attempted in nursing schools around the country, as Kimball and O'Neil (2002) state, "past solutions and traditional demand/supply cycle responses will not adequately address the fundamental issues driving the shortage" (p. 53). Increasing the supply of nurses through student recruitment and expansion of educational capacity is just the begin-ning; it is no longer sufficient for schools simply to provide academic preparation for nursing. Given a 20% average nurse turnover rate in health care (O'Leary, 2002), it is essential that school-industry part-nerships be developed that also focus on retention in the workplace.

STRATEGIC PARTNERSHIPS

"Joining with others in an alliance or partnership is a strategy businesses are using to maximize resources, minimize duplication and forge good will" (Puetz & Shinn, 2002, p. 182). Strategic partnerships are central to successful recruitment and retention and must be based upon a mutual agreement among stakeholders to work together to provide educational and practice opportunities that lead to lifelong and successful careers in nursing. Such efforts must be proactive, coordinated, and collaborative as leaders in nursing—including health care industry representatives, public policy makers, and nursing educators—rededicate themselves more purposefully to creating long-term interventions to ensure an adequate workforce for the future. In short, the educational system and the health care industry share a common goal and a mutual responsibility to prepare new graduates and retain them in a work environment that is conducive to satisfying nursing practice and career development. Schools of nursing must focus not only on facilitating the smooth transition of graduates into the workplace, but also on their retention in the workforce.

To open the dialogue and bridge the gap between educators and industry leaders, schools should consider involving a broad base of stakeholders who share an industry-wide perspective and an investment in the future of nursing. An external advisory group is a valuable yet underutilized resource that can offer schools important advice, feedback, and links to other resources. As an example, the University of Maryland School of Nursing (UMSON) enlisted the support of a Board of Visitors composed of 25 leaders from the community, the health care industry, government, and alumni to serve in an advisory capacity to the school in such areas as strategic planning, outreach and recruitment, technology enhancements, curriculum and program development, and fundraising, marketing, and advertising. The support, guidance, and expertise of this board have enabled the school to advance its mission and attain its goals in the areas of student recruitment and retention. This kind of interchange is reciprocal. Faculty from UMSON serve on advisory committees and boards of community and health care institutions, and work with legislators to bring their expertise to bear on a number of nursing and health care issues. For example, nursing faculty are participating in a demonstration project designed to help a local hospital improve nurse retention through workplace redesign and to assess best practices in care delivery. Through joint appointments of faculty and clinical agency staff, much can be accomplished with respect to addressing the nursing shortage.

ENHANCING THE IMAGE OF NURSING

To successfully recruit students, nursing educators and administrators must work diligently to change negative, outdated perceptions about the profession and enhance the image of nursing. Many high school and college students do not understand the range of career options in nursing available today (University of Maryland School of Nursing, 2001). In early 2002, Johnson & Johnson launched a $20 million nationwide media blitz to boost public awareness of nursing and to attract more applicants into nursing. This initiative, designed in partnership with national nursing organizations, included prime-time television advertising, scholarships, and the development of recruitment tools that are available for use by schools of nursing (Johnson & Johnson, 2002). On a smaller scale, with a gift of $1.2 million from Gilden Integrated, a Baltimore-based advertising agency, UMSON developed a comprehensive, integrated marketing and media campaign to enhance the image of nursing and to reach out to younger students and to men. In addition to branding, advertising, and direct mail, the school utilized focus groups, community outreach, and radio and television advertising to stimulate interest in nursing, particularly among middle- and high-school students. Lessons learned from these coordinated efforts can easily be adapted to any marketing plan.

YOUTH AWARENESS

Because attitudes toward nursing as a career are shaped well before college, recruitment efforts must be expanded to include even the youngest children, beginning in kindergarten and continuing through high school, in order to develop definable career pathways that attract talent to nursing. Nursing leaders agree that developing career interest among young children is an essential long-term strategy for achieving workforce development goals. In a recent article, Bednash (2001) cited the results of a series of focus groups with students in grades 2 through 10 in which children in all grades indicated an almost universal lack of interest in nursing as a career, despite widespread exposure to nursing care and expressed considerable confusion about how nurses are educated. Now more than ever, it is essential that schools of nursing take the lead in clarifying the route to a nursing education and entry into practice. If the intention is to promote nursing as a career destination of choice for young people, then profession-wide agreement on nursing competencies must be clearly articulated, not only within the profession, but also to the public. The U.S. Department of Health and Human Services, through its "Kids Into

Health Careers" campaign, has targeted K–12 school recruitment into health careers and has provided a tool kit of information on nursing and numerous other health professions for distribution in elementary and high schools. This useful information is available at www.bhpr.hrsa.gov.

UMSON began building a cadre of college-bound students who were interested in nursing through public and private partnerships such as the Pre-Nursing Academy, a college preparatory program housed within a city high school. Funded by a grant from the Abell Foundation and facilitated through a partnership with the Baltimore City Public School System, the Pre-Nursing Academy and programs like it are providing more formal links with secondary-school teachers and guidance counselors, thereby expanding student interest in nursing and creating interest in nursing careers through earlier education and exposure. Similarly, legislation recently passed in Florida creates a grant program for school districts to establish an exploratory nursing program in middle schools and a career and technical education program in high schools to promote a seamless transition to post-secondary education and employment in nursing (ANA, 2002). Other collaborative models have been established that include "shadowing" of practicing nurses, mentoring, and "summer camp" programs that allow youngsters to experience the health care environment first-hand (Drenkard, Swartwout, & Hill, 2002).

INCREASING DIVERSITY

Nursing must also enhance minority recruitment in order to build diversity and create a nursing workforce that mirrors the general population. The growing diversity of the U.S. population should serve as a benchmark for the recruitment of a more racially and culturally diverse nursing workforce. Unfortunately, despite this growing awareness, there remains a severe underrepresentation of minorities in nursing and a "mismatch in ethnic distribution between the U.S. population and that of registered nurses" (Kimball & O'Neil, 2002, p. 15). Schools must contribute to the availability of an adequate supply of competent professional nurses at every level and in all needed specialties by purposefully recruiting students from minority and underrepresented groups and providing greater resources and options for career mobility. UMSON has made great progress in building cultural, racial, ethnic, and gender diversity among students and faculty by adopting innovative short- and long-term strategies to promote nursing as a career choice among these groups. With aggressive and targeted recruitment, the school has more than doubled its minority student enrollment, from 15% to 35% of total enrollment within the last decade, and has increased the proportion of men from 7% to 12% during that same period. Minority faculty representation has also grown significantly in recent years, from 11% to 17%. An environment that promotes cultural awareness and provides faculty mentorship and advisement is vital to the recruitment, retention, and ultimate success of minority students.

Building diversity in the nursing population and reaching out to underrepresented populations also includes generational diversity, attracting older students who may be considering a new career in nursing. Until recently, career changers and second-degree students had been a virtually untapped market. Given the current economic climate, accelerated degree programs are quickly gaining momentum nationwide. A recent AACN report (2002) suggests that second-degree students are a captive audience that brings "new dimensions to nursing and a rich history of prior learning" (p. 2). These older, generally high achieving students appear to be more motivated and committed to their studies and therefore may be more likely to pursue advanced degrees in nursing. Employers value the graduates of accelerated programs for their multidimensional skill sets and years of academic as well as life and prior work experiences (AACN, 2002). Although the UMSON offers career-changers who already have a baccalaureate degree an accelerated option leading to the BSN in 16 months of study, other schools of nursing have been successful with even faster-paced programs, ranging from 12 to 15 months. This type of innovative programming should be encouraged.

REDUCING FINANCIAL BARRIERS TO NURSING EDUCATION

To promote access to nursing education, it is essential that financial barriers be reduced through incentives such as increased scholarships, student loans, and other forms of assistance. Schools of nursing should invest resources in raising state and federal aid on behalf of their students and also in fund-raising from the private sector. In partnership with Maryland's premier teaching hospitals, including Johns Hopkins Hospital, the University of Maryland Medical System, and Sinai Hospital, in 1999 UMSON developed a Clinical Scholars Program, an externship that provides financial support for top students who complete their senior clinical practicum with an assigned preceptor at one of the participating hospitals. With almost $1 million raised thus far, the program has been praised not only as a valuable financial aid resource, but also for the intensive precepted experience that prepares undergraduate students for transition into clinical positions in specific areas such as pediatrics, women's health, gerontology, oncology, psychiatry, adult health, and critical care. Upon completion of the practicum and graduation from the BSN program, Clinical Nurse Scholars are offered employment at the participating hospital or other health care institution. The clinical agencies benefit from the opportunity to directly recruit new graduates who are already familiar with a specific clinical area, thereby reducing the time needed for institutional and unit orientation and other in-service programs.

POLITICAL ADVOCACY

In crafting solutions to the nursing shortage, schools must take the lead in advocacy for nursing education in the public policy arena. Such initiatives have in recent years produced legislation at state and national levels. South Dakota recently enacted loan forgiveness programs for nurses who practice in designated facilities in the state, and legislation was passed in Virginia in 2002 making part-time nursing students eligible for scholarship and loan repayment programs. In 1999, UMSON played a major role in the passage of legislation creating the Maryland Statewide Commission on the Crisis in Nursing, which was charged with assessing the current and long-term implications of the nursing shortage in Maryland and developing and facilitating the implementation of strategies to reverse the shortage. The school also joined with other nursing organizations in helping to secure the passage of the Nurse Reinvestment Act (HR 3487 and S 1864). This legislation addresses the nursing shortage by providing scholarships to students, encouraging careers as nursing faculty, assisting nurses in furthering their education, and supporting career ladder partnerships between nursing schools and health care facilities.

POTENTIAL FOR INTERNATIONAL SOLUTIONS

Given the extent of the crisis, international solutions to the nursing shortage cannot be overlooked. In today's global economy, nursing schools must strengthen international relationships by seeking opportunities for collaboration that will potentially generate interest and increase student and nurse recruitment from beyond U.S. borders. This means understanding economic, cultural, and political differences; building relationships; and knowing how to translate American nursing education into mutually beneficial business opportunities. International partnerships that build bridges between local and overseas health care institutions, universities, and governmental agencies can play an important role in expanding global learning and practice opportunities and exchanges, and in strengthening the education and training of nurses who come to American markets. Strategic alliances with overseas partners who may be interested in sending nurses to the U.S. or in replicating the American nursing education model would involve setting up teams of faculty and administrators to travel to such countries to interview potential partners, talk with representatives of health care institutions, confer with government agency personnel, and tap into university resources abroad. Faculty and administrators of UMSON have established such relationships with educational, industry, and government counterparts in China, Mexico, and other countries to broaden the scope of the School's international activities, forge a deeper understanding of approaches to health care and education outside the U.S., and lay the groundwork for future international collaborations in research, teaching, and practice.

HARNESSING TECHNOLOGY

Expanding access to education through technology and building educational capacity via new and innovative ways of teaching are two additional strategies that, if employed effectively, can dramatically alter and improve the "business" of nursing education. Technology has become a powerful, transformative teaching and learning tool in today's information age. Nursing education institutions everywhere are expanding their reach to educationally and geographically underserved regions with the help of state-of-the-art instructional, research, and clinical facilities and programming. Interactive technology, through distance learning, audio-video simulcast, and Web-based courses are just a few of the popular instructional modalities that are enhancing education and training for nurses. In addition to these resources, UMSON offers innovative educational opportunities in its 28 preclinical simulation laboratories, which allow students to develop psychomotor skills through simulated, hands-on learning experiences. In light of a shortage of clinical training sites, this high-tech, self-instructional environment enables nursing students to gain mastery of the basic and advanced clinical skills that will ultimately be required of them in the workplace. At the same time instructional capacity is increased through a reduced need for intensive faculty supervision, thus permitting higher faculty-student ratios in the school's laboratories. A significant portion of the clinical learning and evaluation that was previously restricted to hospital or other health-care settings has been shifted to a safer learning environment, with comparable technological sophistication. Another trend in simulation education is the use of standardized patients: human actors trained to role-play individuals who have specific health conditions. Human patient simulators are a very sophisticated method of clinical education and are expected to become a standard component of nursing education in the future. With virtual computer-generated cyber patients on the horizon, this method in the meantime provides the most realistic laboratory simulation of an actual patient. This kind of experience offers safe learning, practice, and evaluation in the psychomotor and affective domains, and potential for demonstrated improved performance and learning from its use.

DEVELOPING LEADERSHIP AND MANAGEMENT COMPETENCIES

Today's nursing students represent the next generation of nursing leaders. Although clinical knowledge and skills are requisite components of a nursing education, insufficient attention has been given to leadership and management content in the nursing curriculum. Focus groups of nurses conducted by the UMSON corroborate the findings of other studies that point to a lack of nursing leadership and management skills as contributing factors to discontent in the workplace. This suggests that improving the capabilities of front-line managers is pivotal to nurse retention (AHA, 2002). Nursing educators are joining forces with key stakeholders to help advance the role of nursing in the health care industry through programs that enhance leadership and management skills. Building leadership competency in the profession begins with innovative educational programming that rethinks the way professional nurses are integrated into the health care system and how they are challenged, rewarded, and valued as a professional asset (Kimball & O'Neil, 2001). To this end, UMSON was awarded a grant from the Helene Fuld Health Trust to design a course that focuses on enhancing the leadership capabilities of practicing nurses through intensive mentored educational experiences. The goal of the project is to lay the groundwork for addressing gaps in nursing leadership development, particularly for front-line managers. Such programs may serve as a means of increasing nurse retention through more effective leadership.

FOSTERING INTERDISCIPLINARY EDUCATION FOR COLLABORATIVE PRACTICE

Collaborative practice will be the hallmark of health care delivery in the future and therefore schools must foster interdisciplinary education that reinforces the nurse's role as a full-fledged member of the health care team. UMSON has responded to the need for expanded opportunities for interprofessional education and collaboration through an innovative model that promotes clinical and academic partnerships in the classroom as well as in health service delivery. Supported by a 3-year $450,000 grant from the Robert Wood Johnson Foundation, the Collaborative Inter-professional Team Education (CITE) initiative links the University of Maryland schools of nursing, medicine, pharmacy, and social work in the expansion of a prototypical model for collaborative practice through education. The project's central focus is on disease management and the complex health needs of children served by the Pediatric Ambulatory Center, a busy pediatric practice that is jointly operated by the schools of medicine and nursing. Working in partnership with health professions schools across disciplines, UMSON is developing multidisciplinary initiatives, such as CITE and other clinical practice programs to prepare students in nursing to work in collaborative teams within a managed care environment.

Schools must make every effort to identify core content and clinical experiences to foster interdisciplinary education for collaborative practice. Anecdotal evidence indicates that the prevalence of job dissatisfaction among nurses is not only a product of environmental stressors, including inadequate staffing levels and excessive workloads, but also due to a lack of respect and control over decisions and processes required to provide quality patient care. According to Steinbrook (2002), "the perception is that physicians and hospital administrators often treat registered nurses as workers, not as clinicians and peers." It is imperative that all health professionals be educated and prepared to work more effectively as a team, with an expectation that the whole will be greater than the sum of its parts. Enhancing the role of nurses as professional partners could go a long way toward improving patient clinical outcomes as well as nurse morale, productivity, and retention in the workplace. To further advance this effort, the University of Maryland recently established the Center for Health Workforce Development, whose primary mission is to assist health care professionals, health professions schools, public policy makers, and the industry itself in responding to the challenges of educating and managing an evolving workforce. The center will track data, inform opinion, and develop model programs to assist leaders in nursing as well as other health professions in recruitment and retention.

Dealing with Faculty Shortages

An integral part of the nursing shortage is the shortage of faculty. Schools of nursing face a chicken-and-egg dilemma if, as the literature reports, qualified applicants are being turned away from entry-level nursing programs because of the faculty shortage. Budget constraints, an aging faculty, and increasing job competition from clinical agencies have contributed to this problem. Faculty salaries are a continuing issue, and though modest increases over the last several years have been helpful, still higher salary levels are needed to keep teaching as an attractive option for talented candidates, who increasingly are being lured by higher salaries in many clinical and private sector settings (AACN, 2001).

With the slowdown in the economy and the uncertain prospect of any additional state or federal funding, schools of nursing must develop alternative solutions. Consideration should be given to the following options: hospitals and schools sharing the cost of joint appointments of clinical faculty; employment of non-nurse faculty to teach required courses such as pharmacology, information systems management, research methodology, or other nonclinical-specific content; utilization of more master's-prepared clinical instructors; and development of plans that help to increase revenues for nursing schools. For example, the Clinical Enterprise established by UMSON keeps faculty engaged on a contractual basis in active primary care, mental health, school health, and other community-based clinical practices. Reimbursement for services under these contracts is partially redirected to enhance faculty salaries. More schools of nursing should consider these alternatives, to keep salaries competitive and to reduce program costs. Given the aging professoriate, the role of nursing faculty will need to be restructured to help keep older workers employed in educational settings.

CONCLUSION

As Kimball and O'Neil (2001) state, "There is no substitute for enlightened, effective, risk-taking leadership at this stage" (p. 184). It is time to take the lead in identifying opportunities for change, establishing the vision and strategy, and allocating the resources to inspire and encourage that change. By reaching out, developing new partnerships, and making education more accessible and relevant for today's students, nursing schools can continue to provide quality academic preparation while at the same time assuming a proactive role in addressing the nursing shortage. To paraphrase Fagin (2001), as nursing leaders those of us in education must insist that solutions be found to our most pressing problems. We must be seen as part of the solution, *not* the problem, as we build the nursing workforce of the future.

REFERENCES

American Association of Colleges of Nursing. (2002, August). *Accelerated programs: The fast-track to careers in nursing.* AACN Issue Bulletin. Retrieved

December 10, 2002, from http://www.aacn.nche.edu/Publications/issues/ Aug02.htm/ p. 2.

American Association of Colleges of Nursing. (2002b). *Nursing shortage fact sheet.* Retrieved December 10, 2002, from http://www.aacn.nche.edu/Media/Backgrounders/shortagefacts.htm.

American Hospital Association (2001, June). *Trend Watch 3*(2): 1.

American Hospital Association Commission on Workforce for Hospitals and Health Systems. (2001). *In our hands: How hospital leaders can build a thriving workforce.* Retrieved December 10, 2002, from http:// www.hospitalconnect.com/aha/key_issues/workforce/commission/ InOurHands.html.

American Nurses Association Government Affairs. (2002). State Legislature Trends Report. Retrieved December 10, 2002 from http:// www.nursingworld.org/gov/state/htm.

Bednash, G. (2001). A nursing leader speaks out on the nursing shortage: Creating a career destination of choice. *Policy, Politics and Nursing Practice, 2,* 191–195.

Coffman, J., Spetz, J., Seago, J. A., Rosenoff, E., & O'Neil, E. (2002). *Nursing in California: A workforce crisis.* Retrieved December 10, 2002, from University of California, San Francisco Web site: http://www.futurehealth.ucsf.edu/ CWI/nursingneeds2.html/

Council on Collegiate Education for Nursing. (2001). *SREB study indicates serious shortage of nursing faculty.* Retrieved December 10, 2002, from Southern Regional Education Board Web site: http://www.sreb.org/programs/ Nursing/publications/Nursing_Faculty.pdf/.

Drenkard, K., Swartwout, E., & Hill, S. (2002). Nursing exploration summer camp: Improving the image of nursing. *Journal of Nursing Administration 32*(6):354–362.

Fagin, C. M. (2001). *When care becomes a burden: Diminishing access to adequate nursing.* New York: Milbank Memorial Fund Quarterly.

Johnson & Johnson (2002, February 6). Johnson & Johnson launches ad, recruiting campaign to reduce nursing shortage. [Press release.] Retrieved December 10, 2002, from http://www.jnj.com/news/jnj_news/ 20020418_1558.htm/.

Kimball, B., & O'Neil, E. (2001). The evolution of a crisis: Nursing in America. *Policy, Politics and Nursing Practice, 2,* 180–186.

Kimball, B., & O'Neil, E. (2002). Health care's human crisis: The American nursing shortage. Retrieved December 10, 2002, from Robert Wood Johnson Foundation Web site: http://www.rwjf.org/news/special/nursing_report.pdf/

Kosel, K., Olivia, T. (2002). The business case for workforce stability. Voluntary Hospitals of America summary retrieved December 10, 2002 from Web site http://www.vha.com/news/releases/public/02HHsummary.asp.

Puetz, B. E., & Shinn, L. J. (2002). Strategic partnerships. *Journal of Nursing Administration, 32,* 182.

Steinbrook, R. (2002). Nursing in the crossfire. *New England Journal of Medicine, 346,* 1757–1765.

University of Maryland School of Nursing. (2001). Nursing School Focus Groups, prepared by Hollander, Cohen, and McBride, Baltimore.

U.S. Department of Health and Human Services. (2002, September 12). *HHS issues report showing dramatic improvements in America's health over past 50 years.* Retrieved December 10, 2002, from http://www.hhs.gov/news/press/2002pres/20020912.html/.

U.S. Bureau of Labor Statistics. (2001, November). Occupational employment projections to 2010. *Monthly Labor Review,* 57–84.

CHAPTER SIX

Developing an Accelerated BSN Program: The KSU Partnership Model

David N. Bennett, Marie N. Bremner, and Richard K. Sowell

The shortage of nurses in both acute care and primary care settings is a well-documented, nationwide phenomenon. The American Hospital Association (2001) reported that 126,000 nurses are needed to fill vacancies in the nation's hospitals. Dr. Peter Buerhaus and colleagues (2000) in the *Journal of the American Medical Association* predicted that there would be a 20% shortage of nurses in the U.S. healthcare system by the year 2020. It is likely that successful efforts to respond to the nursing shortage will require fundamental changes in the health care system, as well as innovative approaches to recruitment of students into nursing education. There is a need for new partnership models between nursing education, health care organization, and governmental agencies to address this growing national crisis.

The State of Georgia and the metropolitan Atlanta area, like other regions of the country, are experiencing a severe shortage of nurses. By 2010 there will be a 23% shortage of nurses in Georgia unless current trends are changed (Health Care Workforce Policy, 2002). Although these figures represent a significant challenge to the provision of quality health care to the citizens of Georgia, regional economic and social trends offer potential for successful responses to the shortage. A statewide study by the Georgia Healthcare Workforce Policy

Committee on Community Health (2002) documents that economic realities and job losses related to the decline in the stock market and in regional technology companies potentially offer a new group of nontraditional students interested in nursing. Additionally, the events of September 11, 2001, have increased public interest in the helping professions such as nursing.

Recognizing the adverse effects the nursing shortage is having on the health care of Georgians and the state's economy, the governor through the Board of Regents of the University System of Georgia specifically targeted nursing education by making funds available to support increasing the number of nurses educated in the state. An Intellectual Capital Partnership Program (ICAPP, 2002) to support advancement in science and technology in Georgia had previously been established. In recent years, ICAPP funding was used to provide advanced education and industry initiatives to facilitate the development of leadership in science and technology. Due to the economic impact of the nursing shortage, a substantial portion of the 2003 fiscal year ICAPP funds were redirected to provide incentives to encourage innovative partnerships between nursing education and health care agencies to address the nursing shortage. The overall framework for this initiative included the allocation of state funds on a competitive basis to education and industry partnerships that developed collaborative models to increase the number of registered nurses in specific regions of the state. In addition to state funds, the nursing education units and their corporate partners were required to provide resources including matching funds to support the proposed initiative. Using this guiding framework the governor's office sought to leverage available resources to maximize the efforts to increase the number of new nurses entering the workforce in Georgia. Although governmental support from the governor's office and the Board of Regents of the University System of Georgia is a unique feature in the ICAPP, replication in other states may be possible by involving private foundations or other third party partners.

THE SETTING

Kennesaw State University (KSU) is located in the northern suburbs of Atlanta, Georgia, and offers graduate and undergraduate educational programs to approximately 16,000 students from both the metropolitan Atlanta area and the northwest region of Georgia. The School of Nursing (SON) is one of the oldest and most respected educational units at KSU, having a history of providing high-quality nursing education to the region. The SON offers undergraduate, graduate, and RN-BSN programs with an enrollment of more than 300 students. Particular strengths of the SON include the high NCLEX-RN success rate of its graduates, the program's responsiveness to both traditional and non-traditional students, its large number of community partnerships, the operation of nurse-managed clinics, and the stability of the nursing faculty workforce. Even when other nursing programs nationally were experiencing rapid declines in the number of applicants, KSU continued to have more qualified nursing applicants than could be accommodated. This situation was in part due to the faculty's willingness to embrace changes in the educational environment and develop innovative approaches to nursing education, such as using online courses, internships in critical care units or other high shortage/high intensity clinical areas, and mutually beneficial partnerships with local health care facilities.

BACKGROUND TO ACCELERATED PARTNERSHIP MODEL

With a history of embracing innovative approaches to nursing education, in the fall of 2001 the faculty of the SON began to explore new models of education aimed at responding to the region's nursing shortage. Individuals who had completed another baccalaureate degree but now wanted to become nurses were identified as a potential group that could be accelerated in the nursing curriculum to graduate in a shorter period of time, thus increasing the number of nurses available to local health systems. These individuals represented a large pool of mature, educationally savvy students who would bring expertise from a variety of disciplines, as well as valuable life experiences. The challenge for the faculty and SON administration was to develop a model for the proposed accelerated program that maintained high quality and was attractive to second-degree students. An additional challenge was to identify resources to support this program. The commitment by the governor's office of ICAPP funds in fiscal year 2003 to support innovative nursing education partnerships provided a foundation on which a new partnership model for the implementation of an accelerated baccalaureate program was developed.

DEVELOPING THE PARTNERSHIP MODEL

A key component of obtaining the state ICAPP funding to support the model was the development of community and health-care-agency partnerships to support the program financially and to provide job commitments to students after graduation. Based on a long history of partnership with the local health-care system and other educational institutions, the SON was uniquely positioned to enter into a collaborative effort to address the nursing shortage. It was determined that to fully maximize the effects of the new accelerated BSN program, the program would be offered both on the KSU campus and as an outreach initiative. To implement the accelerated BSN program, a partnership model was constructed that included two nursing programs and four corporate partners. All partners joining the collaborative model had the singular goal of organizing available resources to facilitate a program that would expedite an increased number of registered nurses entering the workforce in northwest Georgia.

THE ACCELERATED BSN PROGRAM

In the 2001–2002 academic year, the faculty began to explore a plan to accelerate the progress of second-degree students through the undergraduate program by compressing the curriculum from five regular semesters with intervening summer terms (30 months) to three regular semesters and one summer semester (16 months). Several factors made the accelerated track a potentially viable option for the SON. Community feedback from clinical partners represented on the SON Community Advisory Board indicated a strong interest in the concept of an accelerated track in the BSN Program. Other stimuli for considering the accelerated program included the fact that the undergraduate program has a strong record of providing online education. Fourteen of the 23 faculty members are trained as online facilitators, and the program has been offering online nursing courses since 1999. This expertise provided the opportunity to offer accelerated students a combination of online and on-site courses in their program of study. A final factor that influenced the faculty to offer the program was that at accredited institutions in Georgia, students receive credit for the undergraduate core with the exception of legislated American History and American Government requirements. Second-degree students would only need to take the nursing prerequisites they did not have and the nursing major courses to complete the program. In planning admission requirements, the faculty determined that second-degree students should meet all admission requirements and prerequisites prior to admission to the intensive, compressed track. Applicants are also required to submit an essay addressing their professional goals and their reasons for application to the accelerated track. The top five reasons reported by entering students in fall 2002 for applying to the accelerated program are:

- Desire to help people rather than just focus on monetary gains
- Personal fulfillment of their goals
- Response to events of 9/11/01 and a desire to help with nursing shortage
- Opportunity to take advantage of need for nurses and service cancelable loan
- Interested in improving the standard of health care, even if it is one patient at a time

The faculty determined that an interview would be a necessary step in the admission process. The purposes of the interview were to evaluate the student and discuss the curriculum sequence and the implications of a compressed program of study in terms of work, family, and study responsibilities. A major concern of the faculty was how to handle the student who was unable to complete the accelerated track. They decided to guarantee to the students that they would be absorbed into the traditional cohort of undergraduate students if they had to drop out of the accelerated program.

ACCELERATED CURRICULUM

For students seeking the BSN as their first degree at KSU, the typical curriculum is planned to allow students to take some core courses along with nursing courses. Those students who have completed the core enroll part-time. The KSU undergraduate nursing curriculum is five semesters in length. Students are admitted every semester and clinical nursing courses are taught during the academic year, not during summer terms. The typical undergraduate student will enroll for five semesters with two intervening summer terms. For the accelerated program, the faculty revised this curriculum with the idea of maintaining quality and curricular integrity, avoiding the creation of new courses or a new curriculum plan, and determining which courses might best fit a shortened summer term. The revised curriculum model compressed the baccalaureate curriculum into 3 academic years and a summer term. A decision was made to integrate accelerated students with the traditional students as much as possible to avoid creating additional courses and to promote socialization among the different student cohorts. Additionally, the faculty decided to waive prerequisite requirements for three courses for second-degree students to allow compression of the course sequencing into a shorter time frame.

TABLE 6.1 Comparison of Curriculum Plans

Accelerated Plan Semester	Hours	Standard Plan (no summer) Semester	Hours
Fall semester		**1st semester**	
BIOL 3317 Pathophysiology	3	NURS 3209 Foundations	6
NURS 3309 Health Assessment	3	NURS 3309 Health Assessment	3
NURS 3209 Foundations	6		
NURS 3303 Pharmacology	3		
Total	15	Total	9
Spring semester		**2nd semester**	
NURS 3313 Adult Health	6	NURS 3313 Adult Health	6
NURS 3314 Mental Health	3	BIOL 3317 Pathophysiology	3
NURS 4402 Research	3	NURS 3301 Nutrition	1
NURS 3301 Nutrition	1	Nursing Elective	3
Total	13	Total	13
Summer semester		**3rd semester**	
NURS 3318 Parent/Child	6	NURS 3314 Mental Health	3
NURS 4414 Complex Health	2	NurS 3318 Parents/Child	6
NURS Elective	3	NURS 3303 Pharmacology	3
Total	11	Total	12
Fall semester		**4th semester**	
NURS 4412 Community	6	NURS 4401 Perspectives	2
NURS 4401 Perspectives	2	NURS 4402 Research	3
NURS 4417 Clinical Practicum	6	Total	11
NURS 4416 Leadership	2		
Total	16		
		5th Semester	
		NURS 4414 Complex Health	2
		NURS 4416 Leadership	2
		NURS 4417 Clinical Practicum	6
		Total	10

One example of waiving a prerequisite requirement was allowing accelerated students to take Pharmacology at the same time they enroll in the first clinical nursing course. Table 6.1 provides a comparison of the standard BSN curriculum and the accelerated program curriculum.

PROGRAM COORDINATION

While developing the accelerated curriculum plan, the faculty recognized that students involved in an accelerated curriculum would have special needs for support and guidance that may not be present among traditional students. Therefore, a senior faculty member was identified to oversee the accelerated program, providing mentorship to the accelerated students and serving as a liaison to the community partners. This commitment is one part of the school's contributions to the overall success of the project.

COMMUNITY PARTNERSHIPS

The partnership model formed to implement the accelerated BSN model regionally consisted of six partners (KSU, Floyd College, WellStar Health System, Floyd Medical Center, Emory Cartersville Medical Center, and Redmond Regional Medical Center). The SON serves as the lead agency in the partnership and is responsible for the delivery of the accelerated program.

Since the SON was founded in the early 1970s, there has been a strong partnership between the school and WellStar Health System. Historically, financial support from WellStar has been used to enhance the nursing program at KSU. Most recently, WellStar assisted in the purchase of a sophisticated human-patient simulator that enhances student learning in simulations of assessment and critical care situations. The availability of such equipment in the SON has enabled the school not only to educate its students better, but to serve as a resource for other community agencies. Because of the longstanding collaboration between KSU and WellStar Health System, the initial partnership needed to implement the accelerated program on the KSU campus was undertaken with WellStar. The plan is to offer the accelerated BSN program for 20 students located at KSU in an ICAPP partnership with WellStar Health System.

Based on discussions with state officials and the nursing community in northwest Georgia, it was decided that KSU would expand its partnership model to offer the accelerated BSN program to 20 additional students as an outreach program in the northwest region of Georgia. In order to achieve this goal, the SON partnered with Floyd College, located approximately 50 miles northwest of KSU. Because Floyd College had an associate degree nursing program (ADN), a partnership to introduce an accelerated baccalaureate program for second-degree students provided an opportunity for both institutions. Working with the director of the nursing program and the academic vice president at Floyd College, KSU nursing administration redesigned the initial partnership model to include both Floyd College and three corporate (health system) partners located in the region. The potential partnership model for the region was further strengthened by the sustained focus of KSU president's on serving the northwest region of Georgia, by the number of nurses in north-

TABLE 6.2 Program Partners' Financial Commitment for the First Fiscal Year*

	Contribution (cash & in-kind)
State (ICAPP)	$290,865
Kennesaw State University	$174,470
Corporate Partners	
Corporate Partner A	$54,600
Corporate Partner B	$40,000
Corporate Partner C	$40,000
Corporate Partner D	$25,000
Other Outside Agencies	
Outside Agency A	$100,000
Outside Agency B	$20,000

*This figure represents corporate partners' contributions in actual monies, additional in-kind resources include clinical placements for nursing students.

west Georgia who graduated from KSU, and by the routine placement of KSU students in clinical agencies in the region.

To qualify for the competitive state ICAPP funds, a detailed plan was developed by the partnership. KSU had developed a curriculum model and established a need for the accelerated program that received enthusiastic support at the state level. The corporate partners committed financial resources, clinical facilities for educating students, and guaranteed jobs for graduates as their part of the model. Program partners' financial commitments are shown in Table 6.2.

Further, as part of the partnership model, KSU and Floyd College faculty determined that the best use of the financial contributions of the northwest regional corporate partner would be to improve the on-site facilities, equipment, and software collection at Floyd College. Nursing administrators and lab coordinators from both institutions have been working collaboratively to identify and begin the process of obtaining needed equipment and software. It is the intent of the partnership that an official KSU satellite nursing program will be established on the Floyd College campus that is offering the accelerated BSN program. This proposal is currently under review by the Georgia Board of Nursing.

IMPLEMENTATION OF THE ACCELERATED MODEL

A component of the accelerated model was the involvement of corporate partners in the selection of students. Partners participated in the screening process of selecting 40 students for the program. Admission of the first class of students to the accelerated track has been an exciting process due to the qualifications and energy of the second-degree students.

Demographic characteristics of the first accelerated class are interesting and reflective of the potential of this population of students. The average age for the ICAPP students is 29.75 and the range is 21 to 52 years. There are 38 females and two males. Previous degrees include psychology, criminal justice, communications, business administration, health promotion and wellness, dietetics, and biology. Ethnicity includes seven African American and African students and 33 Caucasian students. Although the majority of students hold bachelor's degrees, one student holds an MBA and another is a retired educational administrator with a doctorate.

Marketing of the program is another area of involvement for the corporate partners. Academic and corporate partners launched a media campaign to portray the profession of nursing as a career path that provides opportunities affording individuals a better life for themselves and their families. An updated recruitment video was produced to target several audiences, including those with a prior degree, men, and residents in the northwest Georgia region, with the intent of raising interest in nursing as a career.

UNIQUE CHALLENGES TO THE IMPLEMENTATION OF THE ACCELERATED TRACK

To produce competent nurses quickly by accelerating progress through the nursing curriculum while maintaining the integrity and quality of an already well-established BSN program is one of the major challenges for faculty and educational administrators. Other unique challenges include the financial needs of students who have limited work options while attending school on a full-time basis; attracting and maintaining sufficient numbers of qualified nursing faculty members; and integrating accelerated students with traditional students who may feel threatened or resentful of students who were admitted into the program after them but may graduate before them.

OUTSIDE AGENCIES LENDING SUPPORT TO FINANCIAL STRESSORS

Students admitted to the accelerated track are typically more mature than the traditional student population, may have family responsibilities, and in some cases are independent from the financial support of parents. In Georgia, second-degree students are not eligible to participate in the Helping Outstanding Pupils Educationally (HOPE) Scholarship Program, one of the major sources of educational funding for

Georgia students. Being ineligible for the HOPE Scholarship makes it necessary for accelerated students to find other sources to finance their education. Students and the faculty coordinator have been proactive in searching for other sources of financial assistance. Two outside agencies enthusiastically wanted to lend their support with this model. Kaiser Permanente, a nationally recognized health maintenance organization, is committed to annual scholarship funding to increase the support for nursing students without expectation of employment commitment. Hospital Corporation of America (HCA), affiliated with two of the four corporate partners, has sponsored scholarships for students committed to HCA institutions. Education and practice partnerships are needed to develop further an increased number of scholarships in exchange for commitment of service.

ATTRACTING AND MAINTAINING QUALIFIED NURSING FACULTY

In order to implement the accelerated track, funding was obtained to hire four additional faculty members and one master's-prepared registered nurse to augment the staff of the Learning Resource Center. An unanticipated challenge was the level of salary required to hire a selected faculty applicant. Due to the nursing shortage, salaries for clinical specialists, nurse practitioners, and other advanced-practice nurses in Atlanta had risen significantly in a relatively short period of time. In light of the rising salaries in practice and other educational institutions and in order to retain current highly qualified faculty, the SON administration sought and obtained increases in salaries for nurse educators at the full professor and associate professor ranks.

INTEGRATING STUDENTS IN DIFFERING COHORTS

A total of 81 students were admitted to the BSN Program at KSU in the fall semester of 2002. Forty of the students are in the 16-month accelerated track and the remaining 41 are in the generic program that typically takes 30 months to complete. Prior to implementing the program, classes were admitted and graduated in cohorts with little contact with students in other cohorts except in nonclinical courses such as Nursing Research, Pharmacology, or Pathophysiology. With the implementation of the accelerated program, accelerated students are admitted with one cohort, join another in the second semester, and in the final semester join yet another. Rumors were rampant among traditional students and some felt that information was being withheld and that the accelerated students had an unfair advantage. The initial strategy used to address these concerns was to introduce the program to the Student Advisory Committee, a group of student leaders who meets with the chair of the SON every semester.

Feedback indicated that this strategy was not fully successful and a decision was made to meet with all students in the undergraduate program to discuss the program and answer any questions they had. Though this did not completely allay concerns, students seemed to have a better understanding of the track and of the challenges facing accelerated students. Another issue was the desire of second-degree students in other cohorts who wanted to be considered for admission to the accelerated track should a student withdraw. Such requests will have to be carefully considered within the framework of this initiative.

SUMMARY

The partnership model used by KSU to develop and implement the accelerated BSN program has been successful. Forty highly qualified second-degree students have been admitted to the program and were enrolled in their first nursing courses in fall 2002. It is anticipated that almost all of these students will be prepared to take the NCLEX-RN examination and enter the workforce in 16 months. Health-care-agency partners are enthusiastic about the program, and believe these new graduates will significantly address the shortage of nurses in their institutions.

The partnership model described in this article represents an initiative that successfully brought state, corporate, and educational resources together to address meaningfully the nursing shortage. Although specific components of the accelerated BSN program and elements of the developed partnership will continue to be refined, the KSU accelerated BSN partnership model has been successfully initiated. The KSU nursing faculty acknowledges that other educational institutions and health care agencies may have different approaches and challenges related to responding to the shortage of nurses in their regions. The KSU model, however, is believed to offer a guiding framework for successful collaboration by other groups in addressing this critical issue.

REFERENCES

American Hospital Association. (2001, June). *Trendwatch.* Retrieved November 25, 2002, from *http://www.hospitalconnect.com/ahapolicyforum/trendwatch/twjune2001.html.*

Buerhaus, P., Staiger, D., & Auerbach, D. (2000). Implications of an aging nursing workforce. *Journal of the American Medical Association, 283,* 2948–2954.

Health Care Workforce Policy Advisory Committee, Georgia Department of Community

Health. (2002). *What's ailing Georgia's health care workforce? Serious symptoms. Complex causes.* Atlanta, GA: Author.

Intellectual Capital Partnership Program. (2002). *Nursing shortage and health care initiatives.* [Data file]. Available from ICAPP Web site: *http://www.icapp.org.*

CHAPTER SEVEN

A Collaborative Effort Among Nurse Leaders to Address the Hospital Nursing Shortage in Cincinnati

Darla Vale, Susan Schmidt, Eugenia Mills, Thomas Shaw, Andrea Lindell, Carolyn Thomas, and Alfred Tuchfarber

T his collaborative effort was designed to develop strategies to improve the recruitment and retention of nurses in patient care positions in the Greater Cincinnati area. Hospital nurses were chosen to be the initial focus because it was believed that the nursing shortage had the potential for becoming a significantly dangerous crisis within Cincinnati area hospitals. The Greater Cincinnati Health Council took the lead in convening the community leadership group and facilitating the process.

THE PROCESS

Initially a group of 43 nursing leaders, called the Nursing Workforce Initiative (NWI), was convened. This group met every 2 to 3 months at the Health Council to discuss issues surrounding the nursing shortage. During the early meetings, the NWI outlined a strategy to systematically address the hospital nursing shortage. The group asked the following three questions: What is known? What needs to be known? What strategies can be recommended to promote retention and recruitment of hospital nurses? In order to efficiently answer these questions NWI members divided into the following four task forces: (a) data gathering, (b) communicating to the public, (c) improving the work environment, and (d) enhancing support of the nurse manager. The task forces met and communicated frequently as they worked on their individual charges. Each task force reported back to the larger group at regularly scheduled meetings.

The first activity for each task force was to conduct a review of the literature to gain a broad understanding of regional and national issues surrounding the focus of the respective group. In order to establish a greater understanding of the issues and concerns of hospital nurses in the Greater Cincinnati community as compared with national data, the NWI decided to conduct a survey of nurses working in Cincinnati area hospitals. Each task force used the survey information to enhance the outcomes related to their separate charges.

DATA-GATHERING TASK FORCE

The Institute for Policy Research at the University of Cincinnati was employed by the NWI with funding from area hospitals to conduct a cross-sectional survey following Institutional Review Board approval. Using the combined literature review of the task forces and the expertise of NWI members, a 22-item questionnaire was developed to provide reliable, timely, and local information. The questionnaire contained both closed- and open-ended items to assess the following key areas: levels of satisfaction with acute-care nursing; factors related to retaining nurses; and factors related to the recruitment of nurses. Approximately 1,000 randomly selected staff nurses from 18 local hospitals received a notification letter from their chief nursing officers indicating that they were invited to participate in the study. Confidentiality of the participants was guaranteed by not associating their names with their responses. The nurses were asked to return a postcard that indicated their willingness to participate in the study. Trained interviewers from the Institute for Policy Research administered the questionnaire by telephone to those nurses who returned the postcard. Two hundred and sixty-nine nurses working in 9 of the 18 hospitals agreed to participate and completed the study. The hospitals ranged from a 144-bed community hospital to a 665-bed university hospital with a level-1 trauma center. The demographic information of the respondents is shown in Table 7.1.

TABLE 7.1 Demographics of Participants (n = 269)

		%	n
Gender			
	Female	96%	(n = 257)
	Male	4%	(n = 12)
Race			
	Caucasian	95%	(n = 255)
	African American/other minority	4.5%	(n = 12)
	No response	0.5%	(n = 2)
Age			
	Less than 50 years	81%	(n = 219)
	50 years or older	19%	(n = 50)
Education level			
	Associate's degree/diploma	54%	(n = 145)
	Bachelor's degree	41%	(n = 111)
	Master's prepared	3%	(n = 8)
	No response	2%	(n = 5)
Marital Status			
	Married	75.5%	(n = 203)
	Divorced or widow	10.5%	(n = 28)
	Never married	12.5%	(n = 34)
	No response	1.5%	(n = 4)
Income			
	Less than $30,000	4%	(n = 11)
	$30,000–$44,999	20%	(n = 55)
	$45,000–$59,999	21%	(n = 57)
	$60,000–$79,000	28%	(n = 75)
	$80,000 or more	20%	(n = 55)
	No response	6%	(n = 16)
Length of years as RN			
	20 years or less	67%	(n = 181)
	More than 20 years	32%	(n = 87)
	No response	0.5%	(n = 1)
Full or part-time status			
	Full-time	62%	(n = 166)
	Part-time	38%	(n = 103)
Number of children			
	No children	45.5%	(n = 123)
	1–2 children	39%	(n = 105)
	3 or more children	15%	(n = 40)
	No response	0.5%	(n = 1)

Survey Findings

Statisticians at the Institute for Policy Research analyzed the data in collaboration with members of the data-gathering task force. Responses were grouped in the three categories upon which the questionnaire was based.

Factors Related to Levels of Satisfaction With Acute-Care Nursing. It was found that 76.5% of the nurses surveyed were satisfied with their current patient-care nursing positions. Of those satisfied, however, 41% were only somewhat satisfied. The remaining 23.5% of nurses surveyed indicated dissatisfaction with their current position (see Figure 7.1).

Two items stood out when nurses were asked to rate the strongest satisfiers with regard to patient care nursing. *Working with patients and their families* was rated highest by 47% of the respondents, and 46% rated *satisfaction of providing needed care* as the most important factor. When the satisfaction factors were analyzed by demographic factors, nurses who have never been married were somewhat more satisfied than their counterparts and the master's-prepared nurses rated satisfaction with patient care nursing significantly higher than

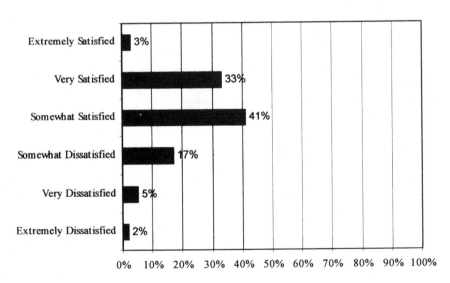

FIGURE 7.1 Satisfaction with Current Patient-Care Nursing Positions.

those with other educational preparation ($p < 0.05$). There was no difference in level of education of the respondents who reported dissatisfaction with patient care nursing. Due to the low sample size of master's-prepared nurses, generalizations from this finding are to be made with caution.

Factors Related to Retaining Patient Care Nurses in the Hospital Setting. Respondents were asked to rate six key items related to retaining patient-care nursing. More than 90% of those interviewed said that the following items were either very or extremely important to keeping them employed as patient-care nurses: staffing, competence, communication, chief nursing officer, workload, respect, and recognition (see Figure 7.2).

When considering a series of salary and benefit-related items, more than 90% of respondents rated base salary and salary commensurate with years of service as very or extremely important (see Figure 7.3).

When asked specifically about what types of things would likely force them out of patient care nursing, the top two responses were inadequate staffing (41%) and intensity of the workload (18%). Providing adequate staffing (47%) and better pay and benefits (24%) were identified as the one change that would increase the likelihood they would stay.

When analyzing whether there is a difference in factors that would keep nurses employed, 100% of the master's-prepared nurses believed growth opportunities and career ladders were important to employment as compared to 35% of associate degree and diploma graduates. Not surprisingly, the master's-prepared nurses also believed salary should be commensurate with education.

Factors Related to the Recruitment of Nurses. Consistent with their priorities of factors to enhance retention, respondents believed better pay and benefits and adequate staffing would draw nurses back to hospital-based direct patient-care nursing. A slight majority, 52% of nurses surveyed, indicated that they would not recommend nursing as a career to friends or relatives. In contrast, only 14% of respondents said they would very strongly recommend a nursing career.

Of the 14 percent who would recommend nursing, the primary reason was *happiness with work/work is satisfying.* Those who would not recommend nursing as a career identified inadequate pay and benefits as the primary reasons (see Figure 7.4). Nurses between the ages of 40 and 59 years were more likely than their counterparts to not recommend nursing as a profession because of the intensity of the workload. Younger nurses, ages 21 to 39, were more likely to not recommend

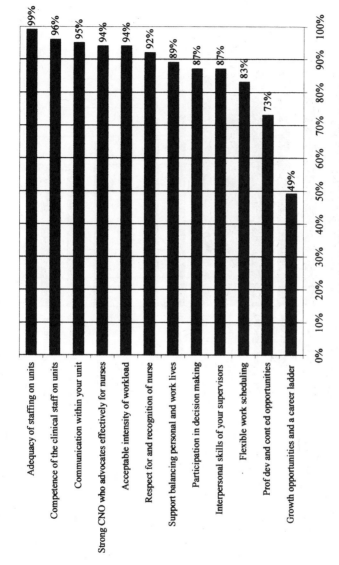

FIGURE 7.2 Issues of Importance to Remaining Employed as a Patient-Care Nurse. (Percentage indicates those who responded "very" or "extremely" important.)

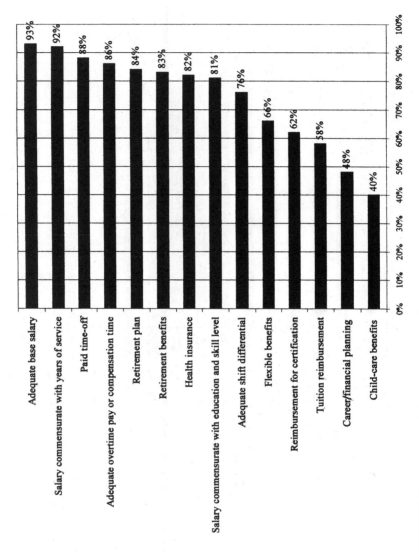

FIGURE 7.3 Issues of Importance to Remaining Employed as a Patient-Care Nurse. (Percentage indicates those who responded "very" or "extremely.")

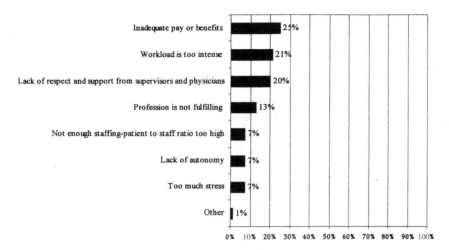

FIGURE 7.4 Most Important Reason for Not Recommending Nursing as a Career. (Percentage indicates those who responded "not very strongly" or "not at all.")

nursing because the profession is not fulfilling or because of too much stress.

After the survey was conducted and analyzed, the NWI discussed the results in a large group meeting. This completed the charge of the data-gathering task force and the remaining three task forces incorporated the findings into their recommendations and activities.

COMMUNICATING TO THE PUBLIC TASK FORCE

The findings from Cincinnati nurses echoed similar national findings, thereby validating which concerns should be addressed locally. The task force on public relations was concerned that 52% of nurses surveyed would not recommend nursing as a career. This presents a bleak outlook when considering future recruitment into nursing in the Greater Cincinnati area. Unfortunately, this is not solely a local problem. The American Nursing Association national survey also showed that 55% of nurses surveyed would not recommend their profession to their children or friends (General Accounting Office Report, 2001).

The first step of this task force was to present major findings from the survey at a press conference. Reporters from the local press and television stations were invited to hear the key results, and a panel comprised of a staff nurse, nurse executive, and nurse educator was available to help interpret the results. The press conference raised consciousness about issues surrounding the nursing shortage and increased support for local and national endeavors to improve the image of nursing.

Task force members initiated a speakers' bureau consisting of nurses who would be available to speak to grade-school and high-school students as well as community groups on a variety of health-related topics. The goal of the bureau is to have speakers reach out to enhance the image of nursing by discussing health care issues of importance to a given audience and by demonstrating that nurses are health care leaders.

The task force also initiated a retreat with hospital chief executive officers, chief nursing officers, and school of nursing deans to explore opportunities to ease the nursing shortage through additional community-wide collaborative efforts. After the retreat, nurse executives from each hospital carefully examined survey results along with their hospital administrators in order to determine additional strategies to retain nurses currently working at their institutions. These strategies included formal recognition programs, flexibility with scheduling, and enhanced salary structures.

IMPROVING THE WORK ENVIRONMENT TASK FORCE

Although findings from the Nursing Workforce survey were not surprising, NWI leaders believed the results confirmed that factors important to the participating staff nurses in the Greater Cincinnati area were similar to national data. A national survey by the Federation of Nursing and Health Professionals (FNHP) found that one in five nurses currently employed plans to leave the profession within the next 5 years (FNHP, 2001). NWI members considered the level of dissatisfaction of participants in this study a serious concern because dissatisfaction is often a first step in the process of changing positions or leaving patient care nursing. The task force recommended several strategies that were implemented the subsequent year.

One strategy was to design a conference specifically for the Cincinnati nursing community. NWI members collaboratively developed this conference, focusing on creating a healthy work environment. The conference offered nurses a chance to revitalize themselves, network with each other, and attend valuable education sessions on dealing with personal and work-related stress. Nurse executives presented awards for excellence to several staff nurses from their institutions. More than 300 staff nurses and nursing students attended the conference.

The second strategy was to enhance respect for nurses in the work setting. Chief nursing officers within the NWI were encouraged to implement a "no tolerance policy" regarding abusive behavior in their institutions. Discussions surrounding this policy raised to greater awareness issues of disrespect. Chief nursing officers also led changes within their institutional environments to create a workplace culture that empowers, values, and rewards nurses.

The NWI was reluctant to discuss salaries of nurses, as others could view this as collusion. After the local survey was conducted, however, salaries were addressed at individual institutions, and survey data provided the rationale for use by the chief nursing officers to improve the salaries and benefits of their nurses.

ENHANCING SUPPORT OF THE NURSE MANAGER TASK FORCE

Nurse manager task-force members reviewed the literature and brain-stormed about the skills and knowledge that are necessary in order for nurse managers to be effective. Task force members interviewed nurse managers at their work sites and asked open-ended questions regarding their preparation for management. The nurse managers indicated that they would like more information on legal issues, mentoring skills, financial factors, employment laws, leadership skills, and interviewing techniques.

The task force developed a series of educational programs to address the identified needs of nurse managers. In addition, educators recommended courses from their institutions for improving leadership and management skills. Deans and directors of six local colleges and universities met to establish a collaborative process for administering course offerings. When possible, the educational institutions agreed to offer on-site programs at local hospitals. It is anticipated that the additional education will enhance retention as studies show that there is a strong correlation between leadership skills of nurse managers and turnover rates of RNs (Murphy, 1996).

RESULTING CHANGES

In February of 2002, the Health Council conducted a follow-up survey with the 18 hospitals in the Greater Cincinnati area to determine if they had instituted changes within the previous 12 months that were focused on improving retention of patient care nurses. The survey found the following:

• Salary—100% of the hospitals increased the base salary for their staff nurses.

• Nurse managers—80% of the hospitals added new or expanded training to their nurse managers in management development or supervisor training.
• Staffing—70% of the hospitals reported that the average number of hours worked by part-time staff nurses increased, with bonuses and increased flexibility in hours.
• Transition—55% developed a new or enhanced program to facilitate the transition of new graduates from school to service. Numerous hospitals established externship programs for junior nursing students in an effort to enhance clinical skills and recruitment after graduation.
• Recognition—40% established or enhanced programs to recognize outstanding nurses.
• Respect—40% established new or enhanced policies, such as zero tolerance policies for abusive behavior.
• Scholarships—35% added scholarships and forgivable loans for nursing students.

The changes in the hospitals have already had positive effects. For example, the staff nurse turnover rate decreased from an average of 9.4% of full-time equivalents (FTEs) in the first 6 months of 2001 to 7.7% of FTEs in the following 6 months. The staff nurse vacancy rate was an average of 11.7% of FTEs in the first 6 months of 2001 compared to 9.9% in the last 6 months of the year. Anecdotal data from 2002 supports continuation of this trend.

The positive partnership experience and increased communication between nurse leaders in the NWI also created some unanticipated benefits. The successful collaboration has fostered an environment where leaders can put aside professional territorialism and concentrate on a shared goal. An educational coalition has been formed with deans and directors of all nursing programs (MSN, BSN, AD, and diploma) to facilitate educational mobility for students and share faculty and clinical sites. The hospitals have provided additional financial support for strengthening co-op programs, student scholarships, and faculty and preceptor support. Hospitals have offered classroom and lab space for schools of nursing to use for expanding numbers of students.

CONCLUSION

The NWI has made great strides because nurse leaders joined and worked together to create a shared vision. As the challenge of providing high-quality care with fewer professional nurses continues to escalate, partnerships between leaders in the community will become even more essential. Leaders must create a visionary master tactical plan to develop a new generation of health care workers and leaders to meet the health care needs of tomorrow.

REFERENCES

Federation of Nursing and Health Professionals of the American Federation of Teachers. (2001, April 19). *The nursing shortage: Perspectives from current direct care nurses and former direct care nurses.* Washington, DC: Author.

General Accounting Office. (2001, July). *Nursing workforce: Emerging nurse shortages due to multiple factors.* Publication #GAO-01-944.

Kimball, B., & O'Neil, E. (2002). The evolution of a crisis: Nursing in America. *Policy, Politics and Nursing Practice, 2*(3), 180–186.

Murphy, Emmet C. (1996). *Leadership IQ.* Englewood Cliffs, NJ: Prentice Hall.

CHAPTER EIGHT

Perceptions of Senior Baccalaureate Nursing Students and Nurse Leaders: A Look at Elements of Success in the Workplace

Rosanna DeMarco and Jane Aroian

S chools and colleges of nursing for many years have placed emphasis on practice-oriented education. Nursing programs are known for the development of integrative learning models that consider the relationship of work realities with academic study. Theoretically, undergraduates are given the opportunity to apply academic learning and integrate it with defined clinical opportunities either embedded in, or offered as, opportunities outside of the nursing curriculum. This chapter describes the experience of a university-based school of nursing on the east coast where there was concern among faculty and administrators that the classroom learning components were being perceived as a separate experience from clinical education. There was little cognitive integration occurring in student experiences. Students seemed to perceive each experience as separate, unique, and part of a program of study that was "clocked off", as if they were just meeting a requirement with little meaningful connection.

Two years ago, the school addressed the "separate but equal" dilemma by examining their curriculum and creating a curriculum map

The authors would like to thank Dr. Joyce Clifford, director of the Institute of Nursing Healthcare Leadership, for her support in distribution of the questionnaire at the nurse leaders conference and to all the students who completed the survey.

emphasizing learning activities that integrated classroom education with clinical learning. A professional development course that had been placed in the middle of the undergraduate generic program was used to achieve this integration. The course was implemented over 10 weeks. Each week, students discuss in seminar format their views about a variety of topics, using specific examples from clinical work experiences as reference points.

One particular week the topic was "Looking in the Mirror" (at ourselves) and "Looking out the Window" (at the professional world in which we live and work). This topic was created to encourage self-reflection because many students expressed grave concerns about becoming nurses. It also was an attempt to have the students think about their future actively rather than passively. Faculty decided to have students discuss their views tangibly as a candid, open dialogue. Students stated openly that in the context of health care workplace turmoil, older and more experienced nurses had been questioning them during clinical and work experiences about why they would want to enter a profession that would "overwork, underpay, and abuse them." This context was used to get students thinking about what qualities they needed in order to be successful after graduation and what they perceived the needed supports could be for them in their transition. A survey was created and students ($N = 16$) answered the following questions:

- What are the professional qualities you think nurse administrators require in new graduates?
- What are the personal qualities you think nurse administrators require of new graduates?
- What kind of organizational culture would empower the voices of new graduates?
- Nursing students talk openly about seasoned nurses being disheartened by shortages, mandatory overtime, and conflicts between MNA and ANA, and they report being questioned about why they are considering being a nurse. What strategies would you suggest that would help you in dealing with these issues of the profession?
- What would you suggest would be practical ways of creating intra-professional alliances?

Prior to the next class meeting, the Fifth Invitational Conference for Executive Nurse Leadership in Academic Healthcare Centers and Major Teaching Hospitals was held in Boston. The conference was sponsored by the Institute for Nursing Healthcare Leadership, directed by Joyce C. Clifford, PhD, RN, FAAN. The institute was created to increase the participation of nurses in health services leadership and promote excellence in policy, practice, and education through inter- and intra-professional collaboration. The audience at the invitational conference was composed of nurse executives and administrators as well as educators from 21 states, Norway, and Canada. The survey was distributed to nurse leader attendees who volunteered to answer the same questions posed to the students but from the perspective of present and future nurse employers. This sample was composed of nurse leaders in a variety of professional positions who were actively employed in health care delivery or education. The sample included executive vice presidents of nursing services, directors of nursing services, managers, midwives, nurse practitioners, educators in academic health centers and academia, and doctoral students in the northeast. In addition to conference respondents, advanced-practice graduate students and nurse leaders from a magnet hospital and a community hospital participated. A total of 62 nurse leaders responded to the survey.

METHOD OF ANALYSIS

Analysis of survey data for both groups (students and future employers of nurses) was conducted by a member who checked for reduction of manifest themes embedded in the recorded written responses (Miles & Huberman, 1994). The analysis team was made up of two nurse researchers and two graduate students. Preliminary data analysis occurred during data collection and through more thorough analysis between the researchers and graduate students. Initially, checking on the accuracy of the students' written comments occurred during a classroom validation exercise. The students worked in groups to confirm that the answers represented were indeed the answers they wanted represented. Data were extracted to identify concepts and categories of specific ideas and suggestions. Identified and validated categories were then brought to a higher level of abstraction by placing all of them on a blackboard and discussing them to elicit central categories. Coding categories began as descriptions then progressed to pattern codes or themes between the researchers. To assure that coding and categorizing was not being "pushed" by the invested researchers, the two graduate students (who were not involved in the study or in the survey process) were instructed in the research analysis method and analyzed the data independently. The graduate students' role was to assure valid representation of the reality of the data (trustworthiness/ credibility) (Polit & Hungler, 1999).

FINDINGS

PROFESSIONAL QUALITIES FOR NEW GRADUATES

Both nurse leaders and students identified three categories of professional characteristics of new RN graduates: (a) values, (b) attitudes, and (c) skills. Students identified honesty, compassion, and advocacy as primary professional values but were also pragmatic in identifying specific work values of team orientation, advocacy, reliability, dedication, punctuality, and hard work. Although nurse leaders identified the same professional needs identified by the students, they added the values of critical thinking, loyalty, commitment to learning, trustworthiness, humility, and moral engagement with practice.

Primary attitudinal themes identified by nurse leaders were "having a sense of accountability," "the impact of economics of health care," and "the relationship between their position and a greater health care system." Students focused on being positive, tolerant, confident, and professional. Students did not identify specifically what they meant by *professional,* but more than 50% of the student group used this term. Both groups identified numerous skills. Students indicated leadership, accurate decision-making, collaboration, versatility, and interpersonal abilities as needed. In addition to each of these skills, nurse leaders added the ability to negotiate, coach a team, be creative, take initiative, be resilient, and avoid judging or blaming others.

PERSONAL QUALITIES FOR NEW GRADUATES

Many of the *personal* qualities identified by both groups were the same values and attitudes identified as *professional* in the first question for both groups. Some additional comments by nurse leaders included a sense of humor, common sense, curiosity, balance, getting to the point quickly, cleanliness, and lifelong learning abilities.

ORGANIZATIONAL CULTURE THAT EMPOWERS THE VOICES OF NEW GRADUATES

Students described the need for peer mentoring and support groups. The majority of the students expressed a specific need for monthly meetings with a designated nurse leader and educator participant where they could express their concerns openly and honestly. Two students suggested that developing approachable leadership was key. Nurse leaders were more specific about suggesting the type of meetings that would allow new graduate nurses to have a voice. For example, orientation programs for each new role undertaken, focus groups, active involvement in advisory groups, and assisting them in creating or being part of collecting survey data related to their professional care experience. One person suggested creating a story-telling forum to increase reflection on the work done in health care organizations. The notions of shared governance or self-governance models were identified less often than the use of preceptorship and mentorship programs. One nurse leader indicated that a quality assurance program directed to novice nurse professionals could be helpful.

BEING A NURSE IN TUMULTUOUS TIMES

Students indicated that direct conversation with seasoned nurses about the effects on them of negativity about to the future of the profession was very important. Several students stated that the focus should be on the philosophical reasons they chose to be nurses, for example, service to patients and families; and connecting with those nurses who share that same philosophy rather than focusing on the health care environment where nurses work. Others stated that they should actively participate in the reform of the work environment. Nurse leaders identified the need to find a positive role model in view of the levels of negativity that exist. Others identified concrete programs, such as reward programs, increased salaries, and increased education programs, for senior nurses who are promulgating the negativity. One nurse administrator felt that a clear message is that nurses are agents of their own destiny, that is nurses should not act as victims, but should be involved in solutions. Finally, one nurse leader encouraged nurses to be passionate about what brings meaning to their work.

INTRAPROFESSIONAL ALLIANCES

Students consistently described the need for individual and group meetings with nurses as keys to openness. All of the students stated that direct communication was a critical element to intraprofessional alliances. Nurse leaders suggested that goal orientation—in the context of quality improvement, health policy, or education projects related to patient care—was extremely important. Others directed their responses to the need to consider diversity and interdisciplinary issues as critical components to alliance building. Specific vehicles that were suggested were the use of journaling, discussions that focused on the commonalities of nursing across specialties of all type of nursing care, and belonging to professional nurse organizations that support professional nurse development.

DISCUSSION

PERSONAL AND PROFESSIONAL QUALITIES OF NEW GRADUATES

Personal and professional qualities identified by both nurse leaders and nursing students were found to be similar. Contemporary professional thought and literature support the integration of personal and professional qualities under the development of life skills applicable to personal lives and the workplace (American Association of Colleges of Nursing [AACN], 1998, 1999; Donner & Wheeler, 2001; Huber, 1996, 2000). Values, however, were only one part of the answer students and leaders addressed when asked about the qualities they thought were required. Attitudes and skills were also identified as qualities needed in the current workplace. The need for dedication, compassion, and honesty on the part of the students was buttressed by nurse leaders, who stated that there is an obligation of individual workers to the institution; that is, accountability and being aware of the relationship new nurses have in the context of the health care system's impact on institutional care. The nurse leaders specifically indicated the underpinning values of loyalty, trustworthiness, and moral engagement with the practice environment as a way of setting the stage to develop attitudes and skills.

Although many students discussed "being professional," the data suggest that seniors (prospective new graduates) identified being positive, tolerant, and confident as key concepts. Each of these attitudes calls for a discussion on sustainability and also the relationship between work worlds and the world of nurses outside of the workplace. To think that attitudes are not influenced by spillover from other systems of influence is naïve and perhaps shortsighted on the part of new employees and employers (Barnett,1994; Barnett & Marshall, 1992). Further, academic and clinical learning organizations cannot support personal mastery without supporting it in all aspects of life. The artificial boundary between work and family does not lend itself to empowerment. A person's work life is naturally connected to all other aspects of life (DeMarco, 1997, 2002).

Both groups identified skills such as leadership, accurate decision-making, versatility, creativity, and resilience as ideally necessary. These skills need to be reinforced and supported over time to allow them to develop. They are also needed to counter the negative reinforcement that may occur in the world outside the workplace.

Although it was anticipated that nursing students about to graduate and seasoned nurse leaders together would represent responses that differ from each other, there was a common realistic agreement in many responses. In addition, nurse leaders mentioned qualities related to organizational commitment. These qualities are highly bound not only to intraprofessional responsibilities, but also to workplace demands. In economically driven institutions that do not necessarily support the ideals of the profession, the participants in this study fundamentally agreed on what is really important when it comes to the qualities that will make or break a successful experience in the workplace. It is interesting that each group identified values, attitudes, and skills that are workplace specific, but did not include their life outside the workplace as influential or connected in any way.

ORGANIZATIONAL CULTURE AND THE VOICE OF NURSES IN THE WORKPLACE

Students and nurse leaders both indicated the need for peer support at a group level and advocated for monthly meetings. Students stated that they were seeking a safe place where they could speak honestly, which was one of the qualities they indicated earlier as important for success. This comment and the one about developing "approachable leadership" suggest that an atmosphere be created where there is no direct or indirect penalty for truthfulness. Nurse leaders suggested forums for story telling, for focusing on issues (focus groups), or for engaging in quality assurance issues. Each of these suggestions is made with the intent of having nurses in practice engage with one another around interpersonal, intrapersonal, and organizational issues; however, they are perceived at the group level where social desirability, politics, and shared dynamics may dilute effectiveness (Roberts, 1997). It is in the survey question related to current nursing practice in the context of tumultuous times (staffing shortages, mandatory overtime, professional organizational conflicts) that both groups discussed the need to find individual levels of support through positive role models.

BEING A NURSE IN TUMULTUOUS TIMES

Nursing students are directly exposed to negativity from seasoned nurses and in some cases they are questioning their future in this profession. Curran (1999) coined the phrase "no margin, no mission" to reflect the relationship between educators (academics) and operations personnel (clinical administrators). Essentially, Curran critiques the lack of integrative involvement of these two spheres of graduate nurse support. This very ambiguity about what these relationships should be perpetuates the conflicts between idealism and realism. It was heartening to find evidence of a reaffirmation of why students and nurse leaders chose to be nurses, namely the commitment of service to patients and family. Yet experienced nurses know that the environment does impact directly on individual perceptions of commitment, quality, and outcomes of care.

Nurse leaders suggested that students find role models and be passionate about what brings meaning to their work versus paying attention to the work environment. Role models are necessary because human beings learn by watching role models (Levi, 1999). Role models share the legacy of practice. One learns to be a practitioner in nursing through education and socialization into the practice by practitioners. This learning involves engaging nurses in ongoing dialogue about practice, research, and the implication of science in everyday care. The body of knowledge of nursing as a practice is socially organized with sets of skills and styles of relating to other practices and to science and technology. This means that learning or doing in the context of practice is never achieved in isolation and the sum of nursing practice is more than its requisite science and technology (Benner, 2000).

Responses to what strategies would help to deal with these real problems for the collective profession are addressed primarily by "find a mentor" and "participate in reward systems" to give tangible benefits to your work. Their responses were insular, not taking into account work environment. For example, it is difficult to know how the individual efforts of nurses will best assist the collective ability of nurses to confront the political economic aspects of healthcare directly (DeMarco, 1997, 1998, 2002; Levi, 1999; Roberts, 1983, 1997). As described by participants, mentorship assumes that mentors are not affected by the negativity that abounds; however, nurse mentors do not live in a bubble. They can, however, reflect a spirit of not giving up and approaching the work environment from the perspective of seeing it as a challenge and commitment. If they are successful in the mentoring experience, how will this lead to success for the collective profession? Is there a place for mentorship at the educational and professional organizational levels without competition and parochialism? Is there a centralized way to engage academics, administrators, employee health, professional nurse organizations in a form of collective mentorship? Does each party to student development have to remain separate and distinct from the commitment to new graduates?

Nursing leaders suggested concrete programs, such as increased salaries and additional education, for more experienced nurses who are promulgating negativity. These are favorable activities that may bring better professional and patient outcomes. More lasting and specific interventions may enable individual nurses to take control of their careers and future as a primary concern (Huber, 2000). Some examples of this include the need to learn and adopt political skills, to increase corporate mindedness, and to engender an entrepreneurial spirit in the context of increasing demands of care (Sullivan & Decker, 1997).

INTRAPROFESSIONAL ALLIANCES

In this survey, nursing students and leaders saw the need for direct communication for alliance building. Both saw nurses as coordinators of care because nurses are responsible for the care of others across health care settings and multiple environments where care is rendered. Nurses have the knowledge and authority to delegate tasks to other health care personnel as well as supervise and evaluate them. Nurse leaders cited the strategy to work with staff on projects to improve patient care and the work environment. Nurses as health care providers who function autonomously and interdependently are also members of a health care team that delivers treatments and services. Nurses bring a unique blend of knowledge, judgment, skills, and caring to such teams (AACN, 1998). Baccalaureate prepared nurses will continue to assume more responsibility for managing health care delivery, involving a variety of delegation skills, case and system management, planning, and integration of care across a variety of settings. This work cannot be accomplished solely in the classroom but in a world of practice in diverse settings inclusive of other disciplinary perspectives (AACN, 1998; 1999; DeMarco, Horowitz, & McLeod, 2000). Alliances within and between disciplines can only be successful when ethical and knowledgeable individuals work in partnerships and with parity along the lines of respect and reward.

CONCLUSION

A number of suggestions are driven by the data presented. One suggestion is a creative approach that has become popular in clinical service, that is, community partnerships. A community partnership with educational facilities, occupational health (from a holistic perspective of health at work), professional nursing organizations, and nursing administration can be created and sustained where mentors can be accessed easily and where commitments to development can be made without artificial boundaries between organizations that appear to deliver products rather than sustain an investment. For example, the creation of a nursing development council could include advisory and work requirements from community nursing professional members related to ongoing development of new graduates. This approach would not be institutionally based and, consequently, would not be insular. Several university schools of nursing and nursing organizations can offer members participation in focus groups, mentorship programs, and quality improvement programs, and would add value to institutionally based education and occupational health facilitators.

Nursing students and leaders do have workplace needs in this challenging and fast-paced health care environment. Strategies suggested to meet the needs are both individually and collectively, based professional responsibilities. This study is an example of how connections are made between workplace experiences, professional education, and the economic realities that surround them. Through classroom discussion, students were able to articulate workplace concerns that threatened their own ideas about their professional choices and possibly their professional future. The survey allowed students to become engaged in identifying problems with solutions. In the same way, nurse leaders were engaged in articulating strategies that are important to future employees. Practice-oriented education in the final analysis means creating a bridge of reality with all members of an education and service team engaged in solutions that are pragmatic and make sense. This collaboration can create and sustain a defined "margin and a mission" for all nurses at and between all levels of practice, formal education, and personal life development both within and outside work.

REFERENCES

American Association of Colleges of Nursing. (1998). The essentials of baccalaureate education for professional nursing. Washington, DC: Author.

American Association of Colleges of Nursing. (1999). *A vision of baccalaureate and graduate education: The next decade.* Washington, DC: Author.

Barnett, R. C. (1994). Home-to-work spillover revisited: A study of full-time employed women in dual-earner couples. *Journal of Marriage and the Family, 56,* 647–656.

Barnett, R. C., & Marshall, N. L. (1992). Worker and mother roles: Spillover effects and psychological distress. *Women and Health, 18*(2), 9–36.

Benner, P. (2000). The wisdom of our practice: Thoughts on the art and intangibility of caring practice. *American Journal of Nursing, 100*(10), 99–105.

Curran, C. R. (1999). Preparing tomorrow's nurses for the no margin-no mission world of health care. *Nursing Economics, 17* (4), 193, 206.

DeMarco, R. (2002).Two theories/a sharper lens: the staff nurse voice in the workplace. *Journal of Advanced Nursing, 38*(6), 1–8.

DeMarco, R., & Roberts, S. J. (2001). [Developing a nursing voice: An intervention study to empower nurses]. Unpublished raw data.

DeMarco, R. (1998). Caring to confront in the workplace: An ethical perspective for nurses. *Nursing Outlook, 46,* 130–135.

DeMarco, R. (1997) The relationship between family life and workplace behaviors: Exploring the gendered perceptions of staff nurses through the framework of systemic organization. (Doctoral Dissertation, Wayne State University, 1997). *Dissertation Abstracts International, 58* 03B.

DeMarco, R., Horowitz, J., & McLeod, D. (2000). An intraprofessional call to reflective alliances. *Nursing Outlook, 48*(4), 172–178.

Donner, G., & Wheeler, M. (2001). Taking control of your career and your future. In *Proceedings of the Sigma Theta Tau International Research Conference,* Copenhagen, Denmark.

Huber, D. (1996). *Leaderships and nursing care management.* (1st ed). Philadelphia: Saunders.

Huber, D. (2000). *Leaderships and nursing care management.* (2nd ed). Philadelphia: Saunders.

Levi, P. (1999). Sustainability of healthcare environments. *Image: Journal of Nursing Scholarship, 31,* 395–398.

Miles, M., & Huberman, A. (1994). *Qualitative data analysis: An expanded sourcebook* (2nd ed.). Beverly Hills, CA: Sage.

Polit, D., & Hungler, B. P. (1999). *Nursing research* (6th ed.). Philadelphia: Lippincott.

Roberts, S. J. (1983). Oppressed group behavior: Implications for nursing. *Advances in Nursing Science, 5*(3), 21–30.

Roberts, S. J. (1997). Nurse executives in the 1990's: Empowered or oppressed? *Nursing Administration Quarterly, 22*(1), 64–71.

Sullivan, E. J., & Decker, P. J. (1997). *Effective leadership and management in nursing.* (4th ed.). Menlo Park, CA: Addison Wesley Longman.

PART THREE

The Retention Front: Promoting Workplace Satisfaction

Intensity and Challenge as an Aspect of Work Satisfaction in an Urban Emergency Room

Bonnie Raingruber and Victoria Ritter

In an era of nursing shortage, when retention issues are of primary importance, it is vital to understand and maximize sources of job satisfaction. Research has demonstrated that satisfied nurses are more likely to be productive (Petty, McGee, & Cavender, 1984), have better job performance (McCloskey & McCain, 1988), and remain at a given hospital for longer periods (Tett & Meyer, 1993).

The relationship between job satisfaction and different variables has been investigated. A number of these studies have examined the influence of managerial behaviors on job satisfaction (McClelland & Boyatzis, 1984; McNeese-Smith, 1997; Tovey & Adams, 1999) and the relationship between nursing practice models and job satisfaction (Buckles-Prince, 1997; Upenieks, 2000). Further, working conditions such as salary and scheduling have been studied as major factors influencing job satisfaction (Mueller & McCloskey, 1990; Tovey & Adams, 1999).

Demographic characteristics, such as age, years of experience, and education have been examined in relationship to nurses' job satisfaction (Adams & Bond, 2000). Personality characteristics of nurses, such as hardiness, have also been identified as influencing job satisfaction (McCranie, Lambert, & Lambert, 1987; Tierney & Lavelle, 1997).

Mottaz (1998) investigated the employee-environment fit by comparing nurses' perceptions of the work environment to their personal values. Pritchard and Karasick (1973) explained that the attitudes and values of each organization make up the personality or climate of that work environment. They emphasized the importance of matching the personality of the organization to the personality of the employees who work there in order to optimize work satisfaction.

Stress has been found to be negatively correlated with job satisfaction (Blegen, 1993; Janssen, de Jonge, & Bakker, 1999). What nurses identify as stressful, however, may be influenced by the unit culture, practice area, or personality of the individual nurse. What is stressful to one group of nurses may not be stressful to another. Therefore, qualitative studies that focus on the ways that individual nurses and units describe job satisfaction are important.

As McNeese-Smith (1997) commented, there has been an absence of studies that have asked nurses to identify the factors that contribute to job satisfaction. The majority of studies have relied on the Index of Work Satisfaction (Johnston, 1991; Keuter, Byrne, Voell, & Larson, 2000; Tumulty, 1992; Williams, 1990), the Job-In-General Scale (McNeese-Smith, 1997), or the Ward Organizational Features Scale (Adams & Bond, 2000), and asked nurses to evaluate the importance of predetermined influences (Williams, 1990). In reality, practicing nurses may be motivated by factors not previously recognized as important enough to be included on standardized, generalizable instruments. Qualitative studies can assist in determining whether or not this is a possibility.

Links have been made between overall organizational climate and job satisfaction (Keuter et al., 2000) but unit level factors are very likely even more important than hospital-wide characteristics. As Adams and Bond (2000) commented, the social organizational unit remains "the most significant focus of analysis when examining nurses' feelings about their work" (p. 537). Although Adams and Bond (2000) concluded that nurses' perceptions of working conditions are a research priority, they examined ward-based conditions, such as ward layout and staff organization, rather than factors such as the unit culture or climate. As Tovey and Adams (1999) pointed out, nurses' satisfaction levels are becoming "more varied due to increasingly varied local work environments" (p. 157). Therefore, studying specific units is of increasing importance.

The current literature would benefit from additional unit-based qualitative studies that allow nurses to self-identify factors that have the largest impact on their job satisfaction. Therefore, the study being report in this chapter was undertaken to examine the lived experience of expert emergency room (ER) nurses in order to articulate their sources of work satisfaction.

METHODS

An interpretive phenomenological investigation (Benner, 1994) was completed that included individual audiotaped interviews with nurses and a 5-hour period of observing each nurse as she or he worked with patients. The nurse manager provided a list of nurses with more than 5 years of experience in the ER. Nurses were selected who had 5 or more years' experience because as Benner, Tanner, and Chesla (1996) reported, expert clinical judgment is most likely to develop after that amount of time working in a given practice area. One of the goals of the hospital in which the study was conducted is to retain experienced nurses. Nurses who had incorrectly triaged a patient in the previous 3 months were excluded. The purpose and procedures of the study were discussed during a staff meeting. Written information and the consent form were left for nurses to review. Then individual nurses were contacted and asked to participate in the study. Fifteen nurses were invited to participate and 13 volunteered.

Approval for the study was received from the human-subject's committee of the hospital. After the primary investigator obtained informed consent, interviews and observations were conducted during each nurse's regularly scheduled workday. Using numbers to code interview responses and maintaining the transcripts in a locked file cabinet assured anonymity of the nurses. After the nurse had completed a brief demographic questionnaire, the investigator observed the nurse interacting with patients and, in the lag time between patients, asked a series of interview questions about the nurse's job satisfaction and practice. The investigator spent at least 5 hours in the ER with each nurse who was being interviewed. The interview questions were asked in an area in the emergency room that was private and the nurse's responses were audiotaped.

Of the participants, 3 nurses were male and 10 were female. Two female nurses were Hispanic and the remaining nurses were White. The range of ages was 27 to 58 with the average age being 35. Years of work experience in the emergency room ranged from 5 to 25, with the average number of years being 9. Interview questions included:

1. If you were orienting a new nurse what would you want him/her to know about the ER?
2. Tell me about the most enjoyable or satisfying part of your practice.

No definitions of job satisfaction were provided; rather nurses were allowed to self-identify what was and was not personally satisfying to them, as is common in a phenomenological study.

The study was conducted in a 500-bed academic medical center with a level-1 trauma center with ANCC magnet hospital recognition. A primary care nursing model was used and the typical nurse to patient ratio was 1:4. Forty-three percent of the patients are from diverse backgrounds; 34% have Medi-Cal, the state-sponsored health care coverage; and 25% have Medicare. The average patient age is 40.5 years and the typical inpatient length of stay is 5.25 days; 41% of inpatients are admitted to the hospital directly from the ER.

Multiple data sources (13 interviews, 13 observations) allowed idiosyncratic information to be eliminated so that consistent meanings could be located as the data were analyzed (Benner, 1994). The whole text and parts of the text of the interviews were read over and over during the data analysis phase of the study. Data analysis that incorporated systemic moving from the parts to the whole text allowed the researcher to check for "incongruities, puzzles, and unifying repeated concerns" (Benner, 1994, p. 113). Participants' reflective comments were interpreted, using the methods of analysis of exemplars and identification of common threads of meaning. After a summary of the common threads of meaning is presented, exemplars will be given so that the reader may participate in consensual validation of the results and decide whether the participants' commentaries support the reported findings (Benner, Hooper-Kyriakidis, & Stannard, 1999).

RESULTS

Experienced ER nurses described liking the intensity of working with complex patients, valuing the unpredictable nature of their work, appreciating chaos, and enjoying the fast pace of an ER because it helped them focus. They appreciated the opportunity to learn from other nurses and physicians on a continual basis. Nurses described simultaneously having a great deal of autonomy and working as a team, and said they enjoyed both opportunities. Nurses emphasized that it was part of their personalities to value intensity and fast-paced, challenging situations by stressing that their home life was in many ways similar to their work life. In exemplar one, a nurse begins to explain these results.

I get bored easily but not in the emergency room. I like acuity. It's a personality thing. Things can and do change rapidly here. The atmosphere is like that old battle cry, "The British are coming, the British are coming." A lot of things are beyond your control in an ER. You can't control how many people are going to be sick on a given day. You have to be able to be alert and flexible. We juggle all the time. It's a challenge to see if you can keep up with everything. I like that.

This nurse emphasized that the ER atmosphere alerts you to prepare for the unexpected and to be ready for whatever might come. She also reflected that it was her natural personality that made her enjoy the juggling and the challenge of the fast-paced setting. In the second exemplar, another nurse used similar analogies to describe the intensity of her work.

In triage it's like you are standing on the freeway telling cars where to go. Doctors and other nurses come to you for everything. You have to have your eyes open all the time. It's like being an air traffic controller. You have to be moving and seeing where each patient will be going and still have a very calm attitude. There are times when you are stressed but you can't be the type who gets easily stressed. Stress to me is when you have four ambulances coming and a code running at the same time and you are the primary person dealing with that. I actually enjoy managing that kind of stress and challenge.

This nurse reflected that she enjoys the stress that is an inherent part of her job. A third nurse commented that the intense pace is something she re-creates in her home life because she feels it keeps her alert and mentally active:

I like the acuity in triage. You know what is going on in all the areas. You control the bed flow. Most of the procedures and cardiac patients are there. You hear more of the stories. You hear what's going to happen to the patient, what the doctor is thinking. There's more action there I guess. I learn a lot by just listening. I think about what I'm seeing and say to myself, "Oh that's why they did that." There's a team feeling. I've changed a lot since I came to the ER. I've become more assertive and sure of myself. You have to be assertive to advocate for good patient care in the ER. The ER has a quick pace and you need to know what you are doing. The pace keeps me going because I'm moving all the time. On my days off I do a lot of things all at once. It drives my mother nuts. She rests. The more active I am, the more energetic I get. It's like exercise for the mind.

This nurse spoke of the momentum of being busy and juggling multiple tasks. She eloquently commented that the intensity is like exercise for the mind; it brings with it a kind of focus and clarity. Csikszentmihalyi (1990) described a similar phenomenon. He explained that flow activities absorb one's attention, require sustained focus, result in greater mental clarity, and bring a sense of joy or satisfaction. Such activities are self-motivating; they contain within them a momentum that prompts one to continue pursuing them. Their reward is intrinsic.

The nurse quoted in the third exemplar commented on what could seem like a contradiction, the importance of both autonomy and teamwork in the ER. She reflected that a nurse needs to make quick decisions to advocate for patients and yet there is a team approach to care. Because one's practice is highly visible, there is a chance to learn from others woven into the quick paced climate of the ER.

A major aspect of emergency room nursing, as described by yet another nurse, is the visibility and team nature of the practice:

> I'd much rather have acute patients because they create focus. We're like a buzz of bees around the bed. We zoom in, fix the person up, and back away. Two or three heads are better than one. Somebody is doing the airway. Somebody is doing the IV, someone is mixing and hanging the drugs. When I first started here I was nervous because of the visibility of everything. It can be daunting. I remember one day all the trauma attendings and residents, and the family of a pediatric patient who had been in a car accident, were watching me start an IV. I kept saying to myself, "Don't miss." Now I like that pace and visibility.

This nurse repeated that the chaos and acuity of the patients demands focus and that is enjoyable. She further emphasized a point made by Heidegger (1962) and Benjamin (1988) that activities shape who you are and how you see yourself. This nurse came to value the visibility and pace of the ER because it had shaped who she was to some extent. As Benner and colleagues reported, sustained practice and experience increase expertise (Benner et al., 1999). Whether practice in areas that require sustained focus further modifies the trajectory of developing skill progression is an interesting question that deserves further study.

Another nurse reiterated that the unpredictable, fast-paced nature of the ER energizes her:

> I like our patients. The variety is such that you really don't know what's going to come in next. I feel really energized when it gets busy. If it's really slow I get lethargic. I love the PM shift because you are constantly on the go. It keeps you mentally alert and moving around. It's like waking up on a day off and having a lot of housework to do. You are ready to go and you energize yourself because you need to. In the ER you just never know when one minute you are perfectly fine and the next minute you have every room full and someone drives up with a gunshot wound.

The variety of patients and the pace of the ER require focus to keep up with the moment-by-moment demands. There is an optimum level of anxiety that facilitates students' focusing on a test or paper that is due because extraneous concerns are ignored. Likewise, the level of activity and the mental alertness required within the ER facilitates focus. That quality may draw nurses to the specialty area.

There are also aspects of ER nursing that differ from other practice areas as another nurse explains:

> When I left critical care to come to the ER the first thing I had to let go of was being in control of my day and setting up my care for one or two patients. Things happen in the ER all the time. You have to reprioritize constantly. I like having different patients, one right after the other. All of us who have been here for a while just know what to do before it has even been said. I can't stand waiting for a certain time to do something like give a medication. I like deciding when to get it done. That's why I like the ER. The pace is fast and there's a lot of autonomy but not a lot of control.

This nurse reiterated a theme mentioned by a number of ER nurses: the importance of being flexible, juggling, and reprioritizing. An important thing to remember is that the atmosphere a nurse has been used to before coming to the ER is an important factor in that nurse's adjustment. This nurse had been accustomed to being in control in a critical-care setting and had to adjust to being more flexible in the ER. He came to appreciate the autonomy associated with that after acclimatizing to the new unit.

The chaotic climate is something another nurse spoke of as contributing to her job satisfaction:

> I like working in the ER because everything is fast paced. We do things boom, boom, boom. We love chaos. The best scenario I could have would be four patients in disarray and stuff flying everywhere. With chaos there are a lot of acute things going on that you can stabilize. I like chaos. It makes you be very focused. You are focused on the patient and whatever the initial problem is, whether the patient has a pulse, whether lines need to be started. You work hard, focus on the problem and get it fixed. I enjoy that intensity tremendously.

This nurse reiterated the fact that chaos demands focus and action. Her comments are reminiscent of conclusions reported by Sobel and Elata (2001) who stressed that by being fully absorbed in the moment and willing to be open to whatever might come along, practitioners develop a sustained attention that results in an ability to see more and notice more of what is happening. The sustained attentiveness contributes to picking up on critical information that influences treatment approaches and patient outcomes. Moreover, sustained attention is by necessity "the polar opposite of indifference" (Sobel & Elata, 2001, p. 90). It is hard not to enjoy activities that require all of your attention and concentration and that necessitate your taking action. Whether nurses whose practice requires sustained attention can simultaneously experience burnout is an interesting question that deserves further study. Are there practice areas that by virtue of requiring focused attention are less likely to retain nurses who feel burned out?

Another nurse reiterated that intense situations demand attention and the appreciation of such a climate is related to personality style:

> I like being in the trenches with several ambulances arriving. I like groveling along, sweating in the chaos. I'd trade chaos for calm any day. I'm an adrenaline junkie. I like living on the edge. Most of the nurses here live everyday life on the edge. Everybody kayaks or mountain climbs or does some kind of extreme sport. We like the unknown, the unexpected. You have to really be alert and pay attention to what is happening during that sort of chaos and intensity.

This participant reiterated that a nurse's basic personality style very likely attracts him or her to emergency room nursing. She described her appreciation in the paradoxical terms of "being in the trenches" and "sweating in the chaos." The terms sound stressful but she reiterated that her perception is that this level of intensity and unpredictability are enjoyable. Her comments are reminiscent of Connelly's (1999) statements that the opportunity to simultaneously experience the order and disorder of life create "an openness to all the possibilities" and an awareness of "all that a moment contains" which helps health care providers notice critical changes and remain open to whatever might happen (p. 421).

A nurse who explained that the environment demands this flexibility also stressed the importance of flexibility as a personality characteristic in ER nursing:

> In the emergency room you can only change the things that are in your control. We can't shut the door. We have no control over our environment in that way. We call the unit and they say they can't take a patient until their nurse returns from lunch. Cat-Scan staff don't call for patients until they are ready. We can't control how many people we take care of on any given day. It's very much organized chaos. But we can go to attendings and get them to help rearrange our world. One of the qualities an ER nurse needs to have is taking satisfaction from what you can and letting go of the rest.

The reciprocal nature of a person-environment fit should be considered when interviewing nurses, especially if the climate in which the nurse will work is intense and unpredictable. Will nurses be happy changing what they can and letting go of the rest in order to focus on caring for the next patient in a busy ER?

A final nurse reflected that she valued the constant stream of different patients she encounters in her practice:

> In the ER there's lots of variety and changeover of patients. You are not limited to just trauma or cardiac. There's a lot of diversity and you don't get bored. It makes the day go by faster. You never get into a rut. You are not allowed to. From my point of view that's good because I don't like to sit around. I like to be kept at a good pace. The ER does that. You see everything and you know everything that is going on in the whole unit. I learn a lot every day and I like that.

This nurse emphasized that he valued learning and the diversity of patients that kept him prepared to deal with a variety of situations. He reiterated that ER nursing is never boring, and that contributes to his overall job satisfaction.

DISCUSSION AND IMPLICATIONS

Consistent with findings from Blegen's (1993) meta-analysis and those of Glisson and Durick (1988), there was greater job satisfaction when nursing roles were less routine and more varied. Manley, Cruse, and Keog (1996) also reported that nurses in their study liked tackling new assignments and learning new skills. Also consistent with the results of a number of studies, nurses in this investigation valued autonomy (Blegan, 1993; Butler & Parsons, 1989; Cavanagh, 1992; Tumulty, 1992) within their practice. It is likely that ER managers would find that job satisfaction among their experienced nurses would increase by rotating assignments between internal and external triage, the resuscitation room, or the child-adolescent beds within the ER so that nurses had an opportunity to tackle new assignments and learn new skills periodically.

In contrast to the findings of Tovey and Adams (1999), working in a rapidly and constantly changing environment was satisfying to the nurses in this study, not a source of pressure or stress. Also in contrast to findings reported by other authors (Healy & McKay, 1999) in this investigation, high levels of intensity and stress were associated with greater job satisfaction. As Lazarus and Folkman (1984) emphasized, one person can evaluate a challenge as stressful while another considers it stimulating and well within his or her ability to cope with the situation. What one nurse perceives as stressful may not be the same for a nurse working on another unit. Therefore, it is vital that nurse managers have a sense of what the climate within their unit is like in order to convey it to nurses who are interviewing for a position. As Johnston (1991) commented, recruitment and retention strategies should be specific to the given setting because there is no approach that is relevant for all hospitals, all units, or all nurses.

The findings of this study are probably not relevant to all ER settings. The complexity and chronicity of patient problems, the volume of ER admissions, an urban setting, the atmosphere of a teaching hospital with ANCC magnet recognition and level-1 trauma center designations, and primary-care nursing model very likely influenced the results. As with all phenomenological results, the findings may be applicable in similar but not all settings. Findings are applicable if others recognize similarities described by the participants as being present in their unit or experience repertoire. Nurse managers would benefit by surveying or interviewing nurses to determine if intensity and varied clinical experiences or other motivations are the primary sources of job satisfaction within their own facilities. It would be prudent to interview both beginning and experienced nurses. It may be that the sources of work satisfaction differ in these groups because the clinical reasoning skills and practice approach of these nurses are significantly different (Benner et al., 1996).

To retain nurses, it is important to determine if the experiences that nurses find satisfying are present in the unit they are interviewing for and whether the nurse who is applying for work is a new graduate or a nurse transferring from another hospital or specialty area. Allowing nurses to spend time on a unit during an extended interview might help them to self-select whether the unit culture matches their employment and personality needs. Other investigators (Consolvo, Brownewell, & Distefano, 1989) have suggested using personality scales such as hardiness measures to encourage nurses to seek employment in fast or slower paced units. Without being so intrusive as to require personality measures, nurse managers can likely assess whether the nurse's personality style is a good fit for the given unit by asking about a "satisfying story" from the nurse's previous practice. If the manager concludes that the satisfying story the nurse shared would be highly unlikely to happen on the unit for which the nurse is interviewing, additional questions should be asked or subsequent interviews scheduled before the nurse is hired. A second interview could be arranged on the unit itself so the nurse would get a better feel for the culture of the unit she or he is hoping to join. Both nurses and nurse managers should take responsibility for determining if the given unit is a good match for the nurse who is interviewing. In this study, an appreciation for intensity and challenge was also an aspect of the nurses' personal lives. Nurse managers might also consider asking one question during an interview about what sort of leisure activities the nurse enjoys in order to assess whether the personality characteristics of the nurse matches the unit culture.

To shift the tide in an era of nursing shortage, it is vital to determine what attracts new nurses to particular specialty areas and to discern what keeps experienced nurses in the profession. Occasionally, staff meetings could be devoted to round table discussions of satisfying stories from practice. Nurses who had an opportunity to hear these stories from other nurses in practice would be reminded of why they elected to work on the unit in the first place and to reflect on what sort of interactions bring them the most joy in their own practice. Scheduling exit interviews with nurses who decide to leave a unit is also a helpful way to learn more about practice expectations.

Further research is needed to determine if sustained focus consistently results in greater job satisfaction, or if this only happens when the personality of the nurse matches the intensity of the practice area. As Sobel and Elata (2001) commented, it is important to pay attention and witness well in health care. Such attention requires intensification, that is, being fully present and open to whatever might happen next. Perhaps in other specialty areas as well as in ER nursing, a stance of being present, focused, and attentive contributes to work satisfaction. Sustained focus may also modify the skill progression trajectory and facilitate the development of clinical expertise. These possibilities should be examined in a variety of ERs and other practice areas.

REFERENCES

Adams, A., & Bond, S. (2000). Hospital nurses' job satisfaction, individual and organizational characteristics. *Journal of Advanced Nursing, 32*(3), 536–543.

Aiken, L. H., Smith, H. L., & Lake, E. T. (1994). Lower Medicare mortality among a set of hospitals known for good nursing care. *Medical Care, 32*, 771–787.

Benjamin, J. (1988). *The bonds of love: Psychoanalysis, feminism and the problem of domination.* New York: Pantheon Books.

Benner, P. (1994). *Interpretive phenomenology: Embodiment, caring and ethics in health and illness.* London: Sage.

Benner, P., Hooper-Kyriakidis, P., & Stannard, D. (1999). *Clinical wisdom and interventions in critical care: A thinking-in-action approach.* Philadelphia: W.B. Saunders.

Benner, P., Tanner C. A., & Chesla, C. A. (1996). *Expertise in nursing practice: Caring, clinical judgment, and ethics.* New York: Springer.

Blegen, M. A. (1993). Nurses' job satisfaction: A meta-analysis of related variables. *Nursing Research, 42*(1), 36–41.

Buckles-Prince, S. (1997). Shared governance: Sharing power and opportunity. *Journal of Nursing Administration, 27*(3), 28–35.

Butler, J., & Parsons, R. J. (1989). Hospital perceptions of job satisfaction. *Nursing Management, 20*(8), 45–48.

Cavanagh, S. J. (1992). Job satisfaction of nursing staff working in hospitals. *Journal of Advanced Nursing, 17,* 704–711.

Connelly, J. (1999). Being in the present moment: Developing the capacity for mindfulness in medicine. *Academic Medicine, 74*(4), 420–424.

Consolvo, C. A., Brownewell, V., & Distefano, S. A. (1989). Profile of the hardy NICU nurse. *Journal of Perinatology, 9*(3), 334–337.

Csikszentmihalyi, M. (1990). *Flow: The psychology of optimal experience.* New York: Harper & Row.

Glisson, C., & Durick, M. (1988). Predictors of job satisfaction and organizational commitment in human service organizations. *Administrative Science Quarterly, 33,* 61–81.

Healy, C., & McKay, M. (1999). Identifying sources of stress and job satisfaction in the nursing environment. *Australian Journal of Advanced Nursing, 17*(2), 30–35.

Heidegger, M. (1962). *Being and time.* New York: Harper & Row.

Janssen, P. M., de Jonge, J., & Bakker, A. B. (1999). Specific determinants of intrinsic work motivation, burnout and turnover intentions: A study among nurses. *Journal of Advanced Nursing, 29,* 1360–1369.

Johnston, C. L. (1991). Sources of work satisfaction/dissatisfaction for hospital registered nurses. *Western Journal of Nursing Research, 13*(4), 503–513.

Keuter, K., Byrne, E., Voell, J., & Larson, E. (2000). Nurses' job satisfaction and organizational climate in a dynamic work environment. *Applied Nursing Research, 13*(1), 46–49.

Lazarus, R. S., & Folkman, S. (1984) *Stress, appraisal and coping.* New York: Springer.

Manley, K., Cruse, S., & Keog, S. (1996). Job satisfaction of intensive care nurses practicing primary nursing: A comparison with those practicing total patient care. *Nursing in Critical Care, 1*(1), 31–41.

McClelland, D. C., & Boyatzis, R. E. (1984) The leadership motive pattern and long-term success in management. In B. C. McClelland, R. E. Boyatzis, & C. D. Spielberger (Eds.), *Motives, personality and society: Selected papers* (pp. 293–308). New York: Praeger.

McCloskey, J. C., & McCain, B. E. (1988). Satisfaction, commitment, and professionalism of newly employed nurses. *Image: Journal of Nursing Scholarship, 20,* 203–207.

McCranie, E. W., Lambert, V. A., & Lambert, C. E. (1987). Work stress, hardiness, and burnout among hospital staff nurses. *Nursing Research, 36*(6), 374–378.

McNeese-Smith, D. K. (1997). The influence of manager behavior on nurses' job satisfaction, productivity, and commitment. *Journal of Nursing Administration, 27*(9), 47–55.

Mottaz, C. J. (1988). Work satisfaction among hospital nurses. *Hospital and Health Services Administration, 33*(1), 57–74.

Mueller, C. W., & McCloskey, J. C. (1990). Nurses' job satisfaction: A proposed measure. *Nursing Research, 39*(2), 113–117.

Petty, M., McGee, G., & Cavender, J. (1984). A meta-analysis of the relationships between individual job satisfaction and individual performance. *Academy of Management Research, 9*(4), 712–721.

Pritchard, R., & Karasick, B. (1973). The effects of organizational climate on managerial job performance and job satisfaction. *Organizational Behavior and Human Performance, 9*(1), 126–146.

Sobel, R., & Elata, G. (2001). The problems of seeing and saying in medicine and poetry. *Perspectives in Biology and Medicine, 44*(1), 87–98.

Tett, R. P., & Meyer, J. P. (1993). Job satisfaction, organizational commitment, turnover intention, and turnover: Path analyses based on meta-analytic findings. *Personal Psychology, 46*(2): 259–293.

Tierney, M. J., & Lavelle, M. C. (1997). An investigation into modification of personality hardiness in staff nurses. *Journal of Nursing Staff Development, 13,* 212–217.

Tovey, E. J., & Adams, A. (1999). The changing nature of nurses' job satisfaction: An exploration of sources of satisfaction in the 1990s. *Journal of Advanced Nursing, 30,* 150–158.

Tumulty, G. (1992). Head nurse role redesign: Improving satisfaction and performance. *Journal of Nursing Administration, 22*(2), 41–48.

Upenieks, V. (2000). The relationship of nursing practice models and job satisfaction outcomes. *Journal of Nursing Administration, 30*(6), 330–334.

Williams, C. (1990). Job satisfaction: Comparing critical care and medical surgical nurses. *Nursing Management, 21*(7), 104–104D.

CHAPTER TEN

Power Sharing: A Strategy for Nurse Retention

Joan Trofino

All leaders are actual or potential power holders, but not all power holders are leaders.

Macregor J. Burns, *Leadership* (p. 18)

Power sharing with staff nurses must be considered an essential strategy if organizational transformation in health care is to be achieved. To revitalize the current competitive health care environment requires a powerful team of participants, including providers at all levels within the organization working together as partners. According to Mahmoud, Lazarus, and Cullen (1992) organizations need to look beyond traditional directive management and the limited approaches of participative management to deal with the challenges of today's global environment if they wish to remain competitive in the local and world marketplace. This chapter examines the concept of power and identifies strategies that will enable power sharing among nurse executive leadership, middle nurse managers, and staff nurses.

UNDERSTANDING POWER

Power is a fundamental need of all individuals. It is at the center of human motivation, and people are continuously motivated toward anything that offers them a greater sense of power and prestige. Conversely, anything that makes individuals feel powerless is viewed as a destructive force. Once acquired, power will be protected and enlarged; it takes exceptional self-control for individuals to surrender their "turf" (Denton, 1997). In today's competitive environment it is essential for all workers to feel powerful, in control of their own performance, and willing to help move the organization to achieve its strategic goals. Yet, accomplishing this goal requires a new approach to leadership by managers and staff.

Managers who are willing to share power with others must demonstrate respect for staff by creating a safe professional environment that permits followers to accept the transfer of power. Sharing power requires redistribution of power from the few to the many. When redistributing power, there will often be fear and resistance from staff and a "push and pull" leadership style from the leader (Denton, 1997). At times the nurse executive leader will need to *push* individuals forward by preparing expert staff nurses to interview, recommend, and hire clinical staff and to further participate equally in the administrative hiring process. Sometimes the nurse executive leader will set an example by returning to school for an advanced degree, establishing new educational job requirements for staff nurses and thus, *pulling* staff toward increased power through academic knowledge building.

POWER DIMENSIONS

Power is exercised in four dimensions. In the first dimension various resources are used to influence the outcome of decision-making processes. Although some first dimension resources are transferred to employees, such as the right to contribute to organizational goal setting or quality improvement practices, the important right to hire, fire, promote, distribute rewards, and control budgets is often retained by the senior administrator (Bernstein, 1992; Eccles, 1993; Hardy & Leiba-O'Sullivan, 1998). Thus, the control for some of the resources associated with the first dimension of power remains with the original power holders (Appelbaum, Hebert, & Leroux, 1999). The power prerogative in this dimension might better be delegated to skillful expert staff nurses who have been educated to interview and hire clinical colleagues. As practice experts, these expert nurses frequently serve as preceptors and mentors, and could easily be prepared in the peer review process to assess clinical performance and distribute rewards. Furthermore, rewards distributed through an agency-wide gain-sharing program jointly facilitated and administered by nurse managers and expert staff nurses would do much to enhance staff motivation, build agency loyalty, and assure monitored quality performance through peer review.

In the second dimension, senior administrators control access to processes that influence decision making. Some aspects of this dimension may be shared with employees; however, strategic planning, an important aspect of decision making, is often "not participative but dictatorial" (Hardy & Leiba-O'Sullivan, 1998; McKenna, 1990). The strategic planning process could easily be included in a power-sharing program by beginning the process early each year and encouraging serious "bottom-up" contributions from all employees. Such a program captures the imagination of all organizational participants, produces challenging ideas, and encourages buy-in by all members of the staff as the final plan emerges.

The third dimension involves the legitimization of power through cultural and normative assumptions (Hardy & Leiba-O'Sullivan, 1998; Hyman & Brough, 1975). The use of the third dimension of power by management increases empowerment practices. Terminology increasingly used to describe empowerment includes words like *team members, coaches, mentors, associates,* and *players.* Increased communication networks help to promote organizational priorities and shared vision among subordinates, peer pressure often becomes more effective than managerial threats, and control is reinforced through the team's efforts and influence. According to Hardy and Leiba-O'Sullivan, workers are more reluctant to call in sick knowing they will have to face team members. Empowerment programs reduce the need to use more visible or coercive forms of power to ensure organizational goal achievement. The stronger such unobtrusive cultural controls are, the less likely that organizational norms will be transgressed, promoting a higher comfort level among managers and a greater willingness to delegate power (Hardy & Leiba-O'Sullivan; Westley, 1990). Managers are able to provide employees with greater access to resources, but avoid opposition by reducing the will or inclination of employees to use their power in an adversarial way (Hardy & Leiba-O'Sullivan).

The fourth dimension of power maintains the belief that practices that promote empowerment could actually result in positive life-enhancing experiences. Empowered employees could believe they are highly valued, feel a greater sense of excitement and passion for their work, and ultimately achieve a more rewarding work experience. According to Hardy and Leiba-O'Sullivan (1998), empowerment may contain a risk of exploitation of workers; however, it also encompasses changes in the organizational environment that may improve the working life for some, possibly all, employees. Such positive work experiences can extend beyond the current work environment as empowered employees gain knowledge and skills that will serve to open opportunities for promotion, education, and exposure to a wider assortment of people and experiences.

An example of fourth dimension power is the development of technology at one acute-care hospital by expert staff nurses. Approached by nurse executive leadership to contribute their expertise in the design of a nursing vocabulary for nursing documentation on a voice-activated computer, expert staff nurses in the operating and emergency departments accepted the challenge. They developed a new vocabulary based upon the medical vocabulary already in use in the emergency department, which they expanded to include orthopedic surgery in the operating room. This effort included expert staff nurses in the emergency and operating departments who collaborated their knowledge building and later served as teachers and mentors to other nursing colleagues. The nurses presented the outcomes of these technology advances to state and international audiences, speaking with pride and appreciation of the part they played in solving the nursing documentation problem by demonstrating a marked reduction of charting time with virtually perfect documentation outcomes (Mulvey, Sowul, & Trofino, 1992; Trofino, 1993).

ORGANIZATIONAL CHARACTERISTICS FACILITATE EMPOWERMENT

Empowerment requires patient leaders who are willing to trust people, have faith in their abilities, and embrace uncertainty. According to Quinn and Spreitzer (1997), four key levers have been identified to assist in the integration of empowerment programs: clear vision and challenge, openness and teamwork, discipline and control, and support and security.

CLEAR VISION AND CHALLENGE

Understanding top management's vision and strategic direction of the organization benefits the empowered workforce by making them feel capable of acting autonomously. Such clear vision communicated through storytelling and stretch-goal techniques by the leader serve to drive employees toward innovation and experimentation as they are challenged to improve themselves as well as the organization.

OPENNESS AND TEAMWORK

Empowered employees must feel they are part of a corporate culture that values the organization's human assets. They must feel that they can work together to solve problems and that their ideas are valued and taken seriously by top leadership. According to Jack Welch (1999) former chief executive officer of the General Electric Corporation, "the way to harness the power of these people is to protect them, not to sit on them, but to turn them loose, let them go—get the management layers off their backs, the bureaucratic shackles off their feet, and the functional barriers out of their way" (p. 144).

DISCIPLINE AND CONTROL

People who feel highly empowered identify that the organization provides clear goals, lines of authority, and responsibilities. They have autonomy, yet they are also aware of their boundaries and decision-making ability. Their goals and objectives are challenging and aligned with the organization's mission and their leader's vision of the organization. This clarity of direction helps to prevent ambiguity and uncertainty and serves to enhance the empowerment efforts. In health care organizations, staff nurses should have a clear understanding of their accountability for ensuring high-quality patient care. Creating work environments that ensure professional practice and empower nurses to act based on their expert judgment is essential to achieving excellent clinical outcomes. When staff feel they have resources, support, and information to complete their jobs, they become more accountable as professionals and more effective in their work (Laschinger & Havens, 1997; Pitman, Laschinger, & Wong, 1999; Sabiston & Laschinger, 1995).

SUPPORT AND SECURITY

Individuals need to feel a sense of support and sincere backing from their bosses, peers, and subordinates. If there is a lack of social support from the various individuals within the organization, employees will be unwilling to take the risk to demonstrate initiative by making decisions and using creative and strategic thinking to solve problems. Instead of acting, employees will seek permission to act, thus slowing down problem solving and their own growth and development. To create an empowering environment, leaders need to demonstrate an ongoing commitment to all four organizational characteristics (Quinn & Spreitzer, 1997).

EMPOWERING LEADERSHIP

According to Quinn and Spreitzer (1997), it is almost impossible for people without power to empower others. Behavioral research has defined two distinctive leadership styles. One is a more directive, authoritarian style and focuses on the task. The other is a more empowering style and is characterized by sharing information, consultation, delegation, joint decision-making, and being focused on employee consideration and development (Vecchio & Applebaum, 1995). Quinn and Spreitzer believed that empowerment is not something that leadership does to employees, but rather a choice that employees make within the context of the organizational environment in which they work.

Employees must see themselves as having freedom, discretion in decision making, and connection to the organizations mission and vision, and be confident of their ability to make a positive impact on the system in which they work. Most empowered people have the following characteristics in common: (a) a sense of self-determination—they are not micromanaged; (b) a sense of meaning—they care about what they are doing; (c) a sense of competence—they know they can perform; (d) a sense of impact—they can influence others to listen to their ideas.

TRANSFER OF POWER ACROSS ORGANIZATIONAL LEVELS

According to Lord and Maher (1991), when power perceptions are patterned and consistent they become internalized models over time. Designated as "power mental models" (PMMs) by Fiol, O'Connor, and Aquinis (2001), the perceptions serve as mental representations of one's own individual or others' power that create predictable behaviors within a selective context. Organizational position, control over resources, and network centrality (individual and group networks) are attention triggers that cause the development of PMMs initially (Ragins & Sundstrom, 1989). Through their model of power transfer Fiol, O'Connor, and Aquinis demonstrated that powerful individuals could increase the power of their teams over time, and as teams transfer power back to empower individual team members. To facilitate transfers, the team must communicate insiders' excitement about the team and its ability to produce results that lead to a new powerful external image. This new powerful image of the team will then cause individual members to be viewed as more powerful, creating a virtuous cycle of power transfers.

NURSING SATISFACTION

A study conducted in 2000 by the Advisory Board Company Nursing Executive Center (as cited in Walker, 2001) revealed that most nurses admitted to decreased satisfaction with their jobs over the previous 2 years. Sixty percent of nurses surveyed considered moving to another hospital position within and more than 40% did not plan long-term employment in their current position, expecting instead to remain in their current jobs 3 years or less. The study also revealed that middle nurse managers maintain primary responsibility for staff retention. A much higher retention existed among nurses who were very satisfied with their nurse managers. A similar outcome was earlier noted by staff nurses who stated during the original descriptive Magnet Hospitals Study conducted in 1981: "We have a high retention rate in our unit but the head nurse is the reason for it" (American Academy of Nursing, 1983, p. 25).

Retention of nurses is the critical factor in achieving quality-driven cost-effective outcomes in health care organizations, such as hospitals requiring large numbers of experienced and specialty nurses. The core or glue of any hospital organization is the expert nurse. New graduates may increase full time equivalents (FTEs) but remain limited in caring for patients with high acuity and specialty needs; this further requires the skills of expert nurses as preceptors and mentors to socialize new nurses into effective professionals. Trofino (1987) described an average retention rate of 7.8 years for registered nurses during the turbulent 1980s when diagnostic related groups (DRGs) were being established as the norm for reimbursement in New Jersey and throughout the county and patients were being discharged "quicker and sicker." It was a time that was highly charged with the introduction of DRGs and the ensuing development of a competitive environment for health care delivery. Those hospitals that were able to boast a low nurse turnover rate and high retention were also able to maintain sufficient nurse power to keep all patient care units open and fully operational. It was also a time when a terrible nursing shortage plagued the county. Then, as now, a survey of nurses revealed that what is most important to a nurse about his or her job is to be treated as a professional and to work in a positive environment where independence and autonomy are encouraged, staffing is good, and flexibility exists, especially in scheduling. Salary and benefits, although listed as a factor, did not preempt the primary drive for self-actualization and independence on the part of the nurses surveyed.

RESEARCH OUTCOMES: SHARED LEADERSHIP

Research outcomes have described a shared leadership model that assumes that "staff empowerment, responsibility, accountability, autonomy, and innovation will result in higher quality patient care" (Spooner, Keenan, & Card, 1997). In 2001, Walker reported the outcomes of a shared leadership model that was in place on a mother-infant unit for approximately 1 1/2 years. Anecdotal feedback seemed to indicate that staff nurses were more satisfied with their practice improvements and work environment. Staff retention on the unit also improved, and increased job satisfaction had been related to the ability of staff to voice concerns and be involved in all areas that related to decisions regarding patient care. Selective elements of involvement in highly empowered environments may also include staff nurse self-scheduling, interviewing, peer review, distribution of rewards, quality improvement, and the ongoing development of quality-driven, cost-effective models for care delivery. Viejo et al. (1999) studied 255 intensive-care staff nurses in four urban hospitals. Researchers examined the direct and indirect effects of nurse-managers' characteristics of power, influence, and leadership style on the critical care nurses' intent to stay in their current positions. Results demonstrated that inclusion of nurse-managers' characteristics explained more variance in intent to stay than did previous research models reported in the literature. Nurse managers with a leadership style that values staff contributions, promotes an environment of information sharing, supports staff-nurse decision making, exerts position power, and influences coordination of work to provide a milieu that supports a stable staff of expert nurses were considered favorable by nurses.

TRANSFORMATIONAL LEADERS' MANAGERIAL PRACTICES

Yukel (1990) identified four managerial practices of transformational leaders: clarifying, inspiring, supporting, and team building. *Clarifying* includes assigning tasks, providing direction about how to do the work, and communicating a clear understanding of job responsibilities, task objectives, performance objectives, and deadlines. *Inspiring* relates to using influence techniques that appeal to emotion or logic to generate enthusiasm for work, commitment to task objectives, and compliance with requests for cooperation, assistance, support or resources, and setting the example of appropriate behavior. *Supporting* is acting friendly and considerate, being patient and helpful, showing sympathy and support when someone is upset or anxious, listening to complaints and problems, and looking out for someone's interests. *Team building* describes facilitating the constructive resolution of conflict and encouraging cooperation, teamwork, and identification with the work unit.

Tracey and Hinkin (1998) asserted that results from their exploratory research highlight three behavioral themes that may help distinguish transformational leadership from effective managerial practices. One theme involves questioning assumptions and nontraditional thinking. This theme includes collaborative problem-solving and decision-making behaviors, as well as behaviors reflective of critical evaluation and analysis. The second theme includes a blend of the individualized consideration and idealized influence that focus on follower development. These leadership behaviors go beyond basic considerations; they emphasize follower self-development and continuous encouragement to facilitate performance improvement. The third theme involves a future orientation with emphasis on " new possibilities," "a compelling vision of the future" and "a strong sense of purpose."

EMPOWERING STRATEGIES

Strategies for empowering nurses include the development of new mental models by leaders, as well as environmental changes on the part of leaders and organizations. Copp (1989) and Trofino (1989) identified the following empowering strategies:

1. Serving as a role model and mentor, giving all nurses the opportunity to copy ideal leadership behaviors as well as the support and guidance necessary to succeed in the workplace and throughout their career

2. Providing opportunities for participation that could include establishing goals and conducting strategic planning sessions with nursing staff, including staff nurses on all nursing, hospital, and medical staff committees; turning the quality improvement program over to staff nurses as the practice experts; developing a professional practice committee dominated by outstanding expert staff nurses who serve as peer review specialists for colleagues; giving staff nurses the ability to offer their opinions to nursing management regarding policies and procedures that affect their practice; and including staff nurse representation and participation at all nursing management meetings

3. Energizing and lending energy, for example, permitting staff nurses to plan their own time schedules and acknowledging their professionalism by trusting their good judgment regarding unit staffing. The role of the nurse manager is to serve as the consultant and to model, encourage, and teach negotiation and cooperation behaviors among nursing colleagues. The leader must continuously seek new vehicles through which staff nurses may creatively express themselves, such as staff nurse educational programs, marketing and nursing research committees, and nursing newsletters. Self- and shared governance

models are also excellent vehicles for staff nurse expression so long as they do not serve merely as a series of councils without ultimate decision-making ability and accountability

4. Resisting the ownership and possessiveness of other human beings (e.g., *my* staff, *my* nurses, *my* patients), encouraging instead individual growth and exploration

5. Remaining consistently sensitive to both the negative and positive effects of the leaders' presence and their words on others. Seek opportunities to commend the staff for excellence. Ongoing honest praise and encouragement from a respected leader serves as a catalyst for continued and expanded efforts toward excellence and achievement and becomes a positive and reinforcing mantra within the organization or department. The leader's presence is always daunting for staff nurses, especially those novice personnel who lack the security that only time and experience can bring. Regardless of the nursing level, the leader is viewed as a power source, or "the boss." Every effort must be made to diminish that perception with nursing staff and, instead, to demonstrate an attitude that is warm, approachable, fair, and friendly. Building trust and communication "across" rather than primarily "down" with staff nurses must remain an overarching goal of all leaders. This effort may be achieved in part through a commitment to a program of walking and talking rounds to all clinical units on all shifts, preferably with the hospital chief executive officer. Meeting with individual staff in the comfort zones of their turf helps to reduce staff fears and tensions in facing the "boss" with their opinions

6. Providing a closer look (depth) by including staff nurses in the interview process for nursing leadership and nursing staff, and respecting their opinions. Use staff nurses in quality-circle sessions regarding unit or department issues, encourage productive problem solving

7. Providing a larger picture (scope), by conducting quarterly staff meetings regarding progress toward organizational and departmental goal achievement with the nursing staff.

QUARTERLY STAFF MEETINGS

Nurse executives should begin with the premise that nursing staff are entitled to information and to inclusion in debate and discussion. Choose a time that is appropriate for most nursing personnel to attend, periodically change the time for the convenience of nurses, and post minutes on every clinical nursing unit. Ask committee chairpersons (staff nurses or administrative nurses) to develop an agenda, lead presentations and discussions, and limit meeting time to 1 hour.

Setting a limit on meeting time and rotating committee reports throughout the year provides an open forum for all participants and also charges the group with the need for concise reporting. Facilitate microphones among the audience to support staff nurse questions, comments, and concerns. This process may also serve as a helpful exercise in encouraging nurses toward greater participation in public policy debates and nursing organizations. The nurse executive leader serves to clarify, expand, and facilitate areas of discussion that enable further insight by staff nurses. Ideally, as the chairpersons and nursing staff gain experience and insight, less direct involvement by the executive leader should be required.

THE ANNUAL MEETING OF THE NURSING STAFF

The annual meeting of the nursing staff provides nurses with a vehicle for organizational recognition. Organizational and nursing department objectives can be presented along with the contributions of individual nurses and collaborative groups of nurses and others toward goal achievements. This meeting should welcome the participation of all disciplines and invited guests, such as local and state newspaper reporters, legislators, and executive hospital leadership, including board members. The program can be easily facilitated with slides or videos recalling the year's events and their conclusion or continuation into the next year.

The development of the annual presentation as a collaborative endeavor among all nurses in the organization further bonds them as one team and permits them to recall with satisfaction those goals achieved. A video of the annual meeting provides an important historical reference and may be used in orienting new personnel regarding nursing's role in the organization. The video can also be shared with board members, nurses or others who are interested but unable to attend. The printed agenda should recognize the annual list of nursing commendations, the results of a never-ending effort to identify all that is great about nurses and the good they continuously offer their patients and the organization. A report of the annual meeting should be published in departmental and organizational newsletters and local and state newspapers. It is important for the organization and the community to gain a better insight into nursing's performance and contributions to health care. Increasingly, physicians are members of multiple hospital medical staffs, providing the consumer (even those within an HMO) with a choice of hospital. The reputation of the nursing staff of the hospital often serves as a strong marketing tool toward consumer choice.

PERSONAL CHARACTERISTICS OF EMPOWERING LEADERS

Empowering characteristics may be found in a wide variety of people and environments. At times, those who empower may not be designated officially as role models or mentors.

They may include parents, siblings, peers, teachers, managers, subordinates, providers, consumers, and even those who would aspire to empowering leadership through literature review and testing. Copp (1989) identified selected characteristics of empowering leaders, that is, open and receptive individuals, excitedly alive with self-confidence, a result of the fact that they had been empowered and are thereby willing to "pass it on" to others.

Empowering leaders are reasonably free from bias, prejudice, and stereotype; they believe in justice and equity. They have resources and are willing to share or enable others to access them; they support connections, contacts, and networks and strive to develop their ongoing creation and maintenance. They are transformational leaders with the primary goal of empowering others to become self-sufficient and free to participate fully in organizational goals and change. Transformational leaders are charismatic and passionate in their beliefs and support an egalitarian spirit within the organization. They respect and value everyone, those within the organization and beyond, such as clients, vendors, the community, the environment, and the world (Trofino, 2000). Personal power is often not sufficient to influence change, but change does require individual characteristics, for example, charisma, an engaging vision, personal values that others would wish to emulate, and an absolute passion to serve as coach and mentor (Senge, 1990).

NURSE EXECUTIVE NATIONAL STUDY

Taylor-Dunham (2000) reported on a national study sample of 396 randomly selected hospital nurse executives. The investigation was designed to integrate Bass's (1998) transformational leadership model, Hagberg's (1994) stages of power theory, and Likert's (1994) organizational climate theory. When staff rated transformational leadership as occurring more frequently on the part of the nurse executive, they rated the work group as being more effective. As staff satisfaction ratings increased, staff effectiveness scores increased; and as staff effectiveness scores increased, staff ratings of extra effort increased. This result supports the importance of transformational leadership as a factor in higher organizational performance and productivity.

The majority of the nurse executives in the study were at one of two stages of power. There were 169 nurse executives (43%) at stage 4 (power by reflection), and 162 (41%) at stage 3 (power by symbols). According to Hagberg (1994) empowerment begins at stage 4. The remaining 54 nurse executives were at stage 5 (14%) (power by purpose; generous and empowering of others), and 10 nurse executives (2%) were at stage 6 (power by wisdom or a sage). None were found to be at either stage 1 or 2. Nurse executive transformational leadership scores correlated positively and significantly with the stages of power. As the power scores increased, the transformational scores increased.

According to Taylor-Dunham (2000), the nurse executives who demonstrated increased transformational leadership scores tended to be in more participative hospital organizations. Furthermore, as the size of an organization increased, the nurse executives were more transformational. Those nurse executives with higher educational degrees also showed higher transformational scores. This study reflects the outcomes of power sharing by a large national sample of nurse executives in hospitals throughout the country. Often it is the nurse executives who have the greatest number of people including nurses reporting to them. Hagberg (1994) established that organizational effectiveness becomes manifest at power stage 4, and yet nearly half or 41% of the nurse executives in the study sample were at stage 3 (power by symbols) where empowerment does not take place. Thus, it seems apparent that a large proportion of nurse executives need further education and mentoring themselves in order to reach the next stage where their nurse executive style includes empowerment, leadership, and mentoring (Taylor-Dunham).

DISCUSSION AND IMPLICATIONS

Taylor-Dunham's (2000) research begins to advance the profile of a highly transformational nurse executive. These individuals would be educated at the masters' or doctoral levels, would work in a large hospital with an organizational culture of participation, and be at power stage 4 (power by reflection, empowerment). Nursing staff, including middle nurse managers, would perceive these nurse executives to be more transformational. Middle nurse managers should model nurse executive behaviors with the nurses, becoming more satisfied with their leadership, with the results being increased retention, effectiveness, and extra effort.

Nursing research increasingly indicates the need for higher levels of nursing education for nurse executives. These programs of study must prepare graduates to assume leadership and management roles in organizations both large and small to ensure the accountable clinical practice of nursing in the organization, and function as a member of the organization's executive management team. The preparation of nurses for administrative roles should therefore include educational experiences in business, psychology, economics, sociology, or health service administration (American Association of Colleges of Nursing, 1997). Furthermore, curriculum designed to prepare nurse executives must include the transformational strategies and approaches prevalent in the literature, for example, mentoring, coaching, encouragement, and power sharing. Hiring practices by hospital administrators should also focus on the need to select only those candidates who demonstrate the educational and personal characteristics most associated with transformational leadership. The candidates must represent personal values and skills that are suitable for the dual role of administrative leader of patient-dominated departments and organizational leader of the evolving professional discipline of nursing.

Increasingly, the profile of the transformational nurse executive needs to be refined through continued research and publications in and beyond the nursing literature. Nurse representatives of accrediting and professional agencies could do much to advance the educational standards that are expected of nurse executive leadership. Educational criteria for nurse executives included in the standards published by national accrediting agencies and professional organizations would assist employers to change hiring practices and raise expectations. If we are to break the cycle of nursing shortages, the transformational leadership style of nurse executives and nurse managers needs to emerge as the expected norm for performance in all health care organizations.

REFERENCES

Applebaum, S. H., Hebert, D., & Leroux, S. (1999). Empowerment: Power, culture and leadership—a strategy or fad for the millennium? *Journal of Workplace Learning: Employee Counseling Today,* 11(7), 1–26.

American Academy of Nursing. (1983). *Magnet hospitals: Attraction and retention of professional nurses.* Kansas City, MO: American Nurses Association.

American Association of Colleges of Nursing. (1997). Joint position statement on education for nurses in administrative roles: American Association of Colleges of Nursing, American Organization of Nurse Executives. *The essentials of master's education for advanced practice nurses.* Washington, DC: American Association of Colleges of Nursing.

Bass, B. (1998). *Transformational Leadership: Industry, military and educational impact.* Mahwah, NJ: Lawrence Erlbaum Associates.

Bernstein, A. J. (1992). Why empowerment programs often fail. *Executive Excellence,* 9(7), 5.

Burns, M. J. (1978). *Leadership.* New York: Harper & Row.

Copp, L. A. (1989). That which empowers [Editorial]. *Journal of Professional Nursing,* 5(4), 169–170.

Denton, K. D. (1997). The heart of the beast: Acquiring and redistributing power in modern organizations. *Empowerment in Organizations,* 5(3), 13–21.

Eccles, T. (1993). The deceptive allure of empowerment. *Long Range Planning,* 26(6), 13–21.

Fiol, M., O'Connor, E. J., & Aquinis, H. (2001). All for one and one for all? The development and transfer of power across organizational levels. *Academy of Management, 26,* 224–242.

Hagberg, J. (1994). *Real power: Stages of personal power in organizations.* Wisconsin: Sheffield Publishing Company.

Hardy, C., & Leiba-O'Sullivan, S. (1998). The power behind empowerment: Implications for research and practice. *Human Relations, 24,* 451–483.

Hyman, R., & Brough, I. (1975). *Social values and industrial relations.* Oxford, England: Basil Blackwell.

Laschinger, S., & Havens, D. S. (1997). The effect of workplace empowerment on staff nurse's occupational mental health and work effectiveness. *Journal of Nursing Administration,* 27(6), 42–50.

Likert, R. (1994). *Profile of organizational characteristics.* Michigan: Rensis Likert Associates.

Lord, R. G., & Maher, K. J. (1991). Cognitive theory in industrial organizational psychology. In M. D. Dunnette & L. Hough (Eds.), *Handbook of Industrial and Organizational Psychology,* Vol. 2, 1–62. Palo Alto, CA: Consulting Psychologists Press.

Mahmoud, S., Lazarus, H., & Cullen, J. (1992). Developing self-managing teams: Structure and performance. *Journal of Management Development, 11*(3), 33–34.

McKenna, J. E. (1990). Smart scarecrows: The wizardry of empowerment. *Industry Week, 239*(14), 18–19.

Mulvey, K., Sowul, M. J., & Trofino, J. (1992). Staff nurses develop voice activated computers for clinical areas. *Nursing Administration Quarterly, 16*(3), 37–38.

Pitman, H. K., Laschinger, S., & Wong, C. (1999). Staff nurse empowerment and collective accountability: Effect on perceived productivity and self-rated work effectiveness. *Nursing Economics, 17*(6), 42–50.

Quinn, R. E., & Spreitzer, G. M. (1997). The road to empowerment: Seven questions every leader should consider. *Organizational Dynamics, 26*(2), 26–36.

Ragins, B. R., & Sundstrom, E. (1989). Gender and power organizations: A longitudinal perspective. *Psychological Bulletin, 105*(3), 51–88.

Sabiston, J. A., & Laschinger, S. (1995). Staff nurse work empowerment and perceived autonomy: Testing Kanter's theory of structural power in organizations. *Journal of Nursing Administration, 26*(6), 42–50.

Senge, P. M. (1990). *The fifth discipline.* New York: Doubleday.

Slater, R. (1999). *Jack Welch and the G. E. Way.* New York: McGraw-Hill.

Spooner, S. H., Keenan, R., & Card, M. (1997). Determining if shared leadership is being practiced: Evaluation methodology. *Nursing Administration Quarterly, 22*(1), 47–56.

Taylor-Dunham, J. (2000). Nurse executive transformational leadership found in participative organizations. *Journal of Nursing Administration, 30*(5), 241–250.

Tracey, J. B., & Hinkin, T. R. (1998). Transformational leadership or effective managerial practices? *Group and Organization Management, 23*(3), 220–236.

Trofino, J. (1987). The mystique of nurse retention and recruitment. *Aspen's Advisor for Nurse Executives, 2*(12), 1,5, 6.

Trofino, J. (1989). Empowering nurses. *Journal of Nursing Administration, 19*(4), 13.

Trofino, J. (1993). Voice—activated nursing documentation: On the cutting edge. *Nursing Management, 24*(7), 40–42.

Trofino, J. (2000). Transformational leadership: Moving total quality management to world class organizations. *International Nursing Review, 47,* 232–242.

Vecchio, R. P., & Applebaum, S. H. (1995). *Managing organizational behavior: A Canadian perspective.* Toronto, Ontario, Canada: Harcourt Brace.

Viejo, A., Boyle, D. J., Batt, M. J., Hansen, H. E., Woods, C. Q., & Taunton, R. L. (1999). Manager's leadership and critical care nurses; intent to stay. *American Journal of Critical Care, 8,* 361–372.

Walker, J. (2001). Developing a shared leadership model at the unit level. *Journal of Perinatal and Neonatal Nursing, 15*(1), 26–39.

Westley, E. (1990). Middle managers and strategy: The microdynamics of inclusion. *Strategic Management Journal, 6,* 337–351.

Yukel, G. A. (1990). *Compass: The managerial practices survey.* New York: Manus Associates.

CHAPTER ELEVEN

STAT! A Four-Step Approach to Nursing Recruitment and Retention in a Tertiary Pediatric Setting

Gail Smart and Anne Marie Kotzer

T he nursing shortage crisis is growing. National supply and demand statistics report a shortage of 110,000 RNs, or 6%, in 2000. If not addressed, this shortage will result in a 40% increase in demand between 2000 and 2020 compared to a projected 6% growth in supply (U.S. Department of Health and Human Services [DHHS], 2001). Colorado is the third fastest growing state in the nation. Growth predictions are for a population increase of 1.5 million people (20%) by 2020 and growth in the over-65 population of 98%. Of the 46,000 nurses licensed in Colorado, 18.3% are not currently in practice (Colorado State Board of Nursing, University of Colorado Health Sciences Center, and Colorado Area Higher Education Center, 2000; DHHS, 2002).

Two factors greatly influencing the future supply of RNs nationwide are the aging nursing population as a whole and the aging nursing faculty. Currently in Colorado, the mean age of RNs is 47 years, with 75% of RNs over 41 years of age. The mean age of Colorado nursing faculty is 51 years. In a recent survey, 17% of Colorado nurses do not expect to be practicing in 5 years and 27.8% are uncertain about whether they will remain in nursing (Colorado State Board of Nursing et al., 2000).

The current shortage is different from previous shortages in several ways. In addition to the aging population, there are fewer young people entering the workforce, and the racial and ethnic makeup of the current workforce does not reflect the increasing diversity of the United States. As well, the younger generation perceives nursing as unappealing, and fewer resources and greater demands have resulted in dissatisfaction among nurses (Hopkins, 2001; Kimball & O'Neil, 2002).

The nursing shortage poses inadequate staffing levels and increases patient safety risks. Nationally, inadequate staffing levels have been a factor in 24% of the 1,609 sentinel events reported by the Joint Commission on Accreditation of Healthcare Organization, (2002). A recent study reports that sufficient staffing is associated with a shorter length of stay and lower rates of urinary tract infections and upper gastrointestinal bleeding among hospitalized medical patients. Lower rates of other comorbidities, such as pneumonia, shock or cardiac arrest, sepsis, and deep venous thromboses also were associated with a higher proportion of hours of care provided by RNs (Needleman, Buerhaus, Mattke, Stewart, & Zelevinsky, 2002).

Adequate staffing is a significant factor contributing to the satisfaction of nurses and it is a primary motivator for nurses making employment choices. According to the Healthcare Information Resource Center (1998) nursing shortage study, nursing managers, registered nurses, and licensed practical nurses cited an insufficient supply of qualified managers or experienced staff as the most likely reason for the current shortage.

Hiring nurses with additional educational requirements or specialty practice, such as critical care, surgical, or pediatric experience, compounds the recruiting challenge. It is essential that adequate supplies of competent nurses be available to meet the increasingly complex patient care needs. In response to our increasing local population, aging of the nursing workforce, increased patient acuity level, and the state-required BSN degree for entry into practice, a comprehensive recruitment and retention strategy was implemented at The Children's Hospital in Denver.

ADDRESSING THE SHORTAGE

SHORT-TERM STRATEGIES

One short-term strategy to addressing the shortage is the recruitment of foreign nurses. Though international staffing agencies are eager to assist in the placement of foreign nurses, they often require fees as high as 35% of the nurse's first year salary (J. Nelly, personal communication, November, 2001; C. P. Stanton, personal communication, July

30, 2001). High costs, lengthy immigration processes, language barriers, and cultural differences can be huge challenges to the recruitment and retention of foreign staff (Peterson, 2001). Last, and possibly most important, is that this approach poses serious questions from an ethical perspective, because the nursing shortage is international in scope.

It has been our experience that short-term strategies to remedy the nursing shortage have limitations. Monetary sign-on bonuses initially can be helpful to recruit nurses, but they quickly deteriorate the morale and internal equity of existing staff. This approach also becomes increasingly expensive and often results in "hospital-shopping" on the part of nurses. With hospitals operating under tight profit margins, monetary bonuses increase the already high cost of turnover. An internal employee opinion survey at our hospital showed that although improving RN compensation was an important factor to recruitment, salaries were not the only important benefit to a nurse when considering a new job. Strategies that focus on more sustainable solutions to the nursing shortage were recommended.

LONG-TERM STRATEGIES

National reports from nursing organizations, associations, panels, coalitions, consortiums, and government entities have devised a wide variety of long-term recommendations with primarily the same theme. To increase the supply of nurses, we need more effective recruitment, expanded educational opportunities and career options, improved compensation, increased visibility of nurses' contributions to the quality of health care, strong nursing leadership, and a regard for nurses as strategic assets in the work environment (American Hospital Association, 2001; Kimball & O'Neil, 2002; Peterson, 2001). The purpose of this chapter is to describe a four-step approach to nursing recruitment and retention that was developed and implemented at The Children's Hospital (TCH) in Denver. This approach incorporates both short-term and long-term strategies to address the shortage in this institution.

THE CHILDREN'S HOSPITAL APPROACH

With support from senior management, human resources, and the division of nursing, TCH proactively prepared for the times ahead as they hired an advanced practice nurse in 2000 to recruit and retain qualified nurses for the organization. Since that time, the four-step approach, STAT! (Student and Employee Recruitment, Teaching the Specialty, Active Mentorship, and Time to Listen), has been underway to help address the needs stemming from the nursing shortage. The acronym STAT also denotes the urgency and significance of the current crisis and the need for immediate intervention to address this critical healthcare problem.

Step One: Student and Employee Recruitment

The Children's Hospital has created several programs to attract Denver area elementary- and secondary-school students into a career in health care, specifically nursing. The Medical Career Collaborative (MC^2) represents a partnership between TCH, Manual High School, and the University of Colorado Health Sciences Center. Created to promote an awareness of health care career opportunities among low-income high-school students, this program combines advanced classes, including college courses, with job shadowing and paid internships within the hospital.

Since its inception in 1999, 20 students have graduated from the MC^2 program. A longitudinal study is being conducted to follow these graduates following their secondary education. To date, 9 of the 12 students responding to a postgraduation survey indicated that they are currently enrolled in college or a technical school. Although too early in their college courses to say definitively, students have expressed interest in the following: nursing, radiology, environmental biology, fire fighting and EMT, general pediatrics, and psychology.

Another newly created program that is aimed at attracting high-school students into nursing is Spend a Day with a Children's Hospital Nurse. This 6-hour career day, offered several times per year, consists of unit-based hospital tours, a question and answer session with nurses, and a video about pediatric nursing. The students get real-life hands-on experience by taking blood pressures, handling operating room (OR) equipment, wearing OR protective clothing, starting intravenous lines on mannequins, and participating in mock codes with mannequins. In addition to educating high-schools students about opportunities in nursing, the career days share valuable information with school counselors, who in turn can reinforce and share the information with their students to assist them better in planning for a nursing career.

Over the past year and a half, 123 students and 30 high-school counselors from 26 area schools have participated in the program. Prior to participating in the nursing career day, 50 students reported never having had a conversation about nursing as a career choice.

Results of a survey completed by students at the end of the day at the hospital indicated that 55 of the 123 students were *very interested,* and 49 were *somewhat interested* in pursuing nursing as a profession. One initial indicator of success of this program is that a counselor enrolled in a nursing degree program.

Another example of the career-day model is the collaboration of TCH with the Colorado UpLIFT Program. In conjunction with the Boy Scouts of America, Colorado UpLIFT coordinates career fairs in 12 urban schools. The purpose of the career fair activity is to get elementary- and middle-school students excited about options for their future by exposing them to a variety of careers. This program mentors students to promote positive attitude, lifestyle, and career choices. The fairs are designed to introduce students to six or seven different career opportunities. During each career fair, approximately 15 presenters in one room share 6- to 7-minute information sessions with rotating groups of students. Feedback from students has been positive and they reported having gained new insights about the diverse field of nursing.

In July 2001, TCH organized a non-nursing employee career day to attract and recruit current non-nurse employees into a career in nursing. Representatives from five associate and baccalaureate-degree nursing programs in the Denver metropolitan area were on-site to answer employee's questions and to share specific curricula. Forty TCH staff from 25 different departments attended the career day. At the time of this writing, five employees had enrolled in a nursing program. This program encouraged non-nursing staff to change careers while maintaining current employment in their respective departments, preserving their seniority, and qualifying for additional tuition assistance through a recently created pilot program. Under this program, a 1-year commitment of full-time employment is required for each year of funding, up to a maximum of 5 years. Funds can be used for tuition, books, and fees. More than 20 employees applied for this special tuition assistance. A database will be created to track the outcomes of recruitment and retention.

In 2002, The Children's Hospital received funding from the Denver Mayor's Office of Workforce Development to establish a cooperative education program. The purpose of the Mayor's Workforce grant is to assist Denver businesses in obtaining and retaining qualified workers while upgrading the skills of current employees. Two training programs have been established: Basic Skills and Upgrade Training. TCH utilizes these funds to pay for the following classes: Sterile Processing certificate program, Medical Terminology, Food Services, and Spanish. To qualify, the employer must agree to match funding dollar-for-dollar up to $50,000 for a 1-year period. Potential program benefits include a better-trained workforce, increased retention of employees, and the potential to earn a higher working wage. At the time of this writing, 49 trainees participated in the program and were still employed at our hospital.

STEP TWO: TEACHING THE SPECIALTY

Through clinical rotations and specialty courses, students who have chosen a career in nursing but have not yet decided on pediatrics as a specialty are provided with various levels of on-the-job training opportunities to encourage them to choose pediatrics, and TCH, as their specialty focus. Two roles, the clinical technician and the clinical assistant, were created to assist nursing students in learning the specialty of pediatrics. One requirement for employment in the clinical technician role is enrollment in a BSN, nursing doctorate (ND), or pre-med program. The clinical assistant position requires completion of the junior BSN year or ND medical/surgical clinical rotation, with completion of the pediatric rotation preferred. These paid positions afford on-the-job training while supporting the unit-based nurses who often become occupied with nonprofessional tasks.

The orientation for clinical technicians is conducted on the inpatient unit by professional nursing staff. A primary focus of the orientation is to explain how the pediatric patient population differs from caring for adults, that is, that children are not just little adults. Concepts of family-centered care are emphasized as well as how to incorporate this philosophy into interactions with patients and families. Responsibilities of the clinical technician include unit stocking, cleaning equipment, preparing rooms for admissions and discharges, and transporting patients. Clinical technician competencies were developed and serve as the guidelines for job performance evaluation. Between 2001 and 2002, eight clinical technicians were hired at our organization.

In contrast, the clinical assistant can perform basic level patient care skills such as obtaining vital signs, oral/nasal/tracheal suctioning, assisting with activities of daily living, and special procedures under the direct supervision of a registered nurse (RN). Orientation classes for this population are offered six times per year and contain content similar to the RN orientation, including a review of policies and procedures, references of care, professional expectations, ethical issues, and patient rights. Other classes incorporate concepts related to caring for the dying child, recognition of child abuse or neglect, family-centered care, and age-specific developmental care. Clinical assistants are also taught to identify from baseline significant changes in neurological, cardiovascular, renal, and respiratory status specific to the pediatric population.

An added variation of the clinical assistant role is a "flex" clinical assistant, which requires completion of the ND or BSN pediatric clinical rotation. The flex clinical assistant can float to medical and surgical units within the hospital after unit-specific orientation to gain a broader range of clinical experiences. Shifts and hours per week required for both the clinical technician and clinical assistant roles are flexible in order to accommodate the students' varying schedules. In the past 3 years, 90 students have been hired as flex and 60 as unit-based clinical assistants.

Typically, schools of nursing provide instructors to supervise students in clinical rotations within various clinical settings. Several years ago, TCH collaborated with a BSN nursing program to develop a unique model for precepting nursing students known as the Clinical Teaching Associate (CTA) model. Criteria for CTA selection include a minimum of 2 years' pediatric experience (clinical level III status), excellent communication skills as demonstrated through performance evaluations, and a desire to teach. Each CTA is encouraged to attend a preceptor workshop prior to the clinical rotation. Weekly for 6 weeks, each CTA precepts one or two students for a 12-hour shift. The student has his or her own assignment with close supervision of direct patient care provided by a consistent CTA for the entire rotation. Besides the CTA, a clinical faculty (CF) member provides support to students. CFs are TCH-employed master's-prepared nurses with responsibilities for mentoring student learners. CFs review students' written assignments, facilitate group clinical conferences, evaluate student performance, and provide leadership related to topics such as family-centered care, evidence-based practice, and ethics.

During 2001, TCH placed 218 students in clinical experiences for a total of 18,671 hours of instruction. With the high demand from schools for more student placements, TCH committed to providing clinical rotations, preceptors, and clinical faculty for additional nursing students in 2002. These experiences in the clinical setting have been invaluable to the students' understanding of, and appreciation for, the pediatric patient population. As a result of their positive experiences in the clinical setting, approximately 30 to 40 students are hired as new graduate nurses each year. In 2001 alone, TCH hired 54 new graduate nurses. Survey data showed that 36% of the new graduate hires directly related their desire to work at TCH to a positive clinical rotation as a student.

Students and faculty realize that additional opportunities in the pediatric clinical setting are necessary to provide a better understanding of the specialty. Most students are placed on acute rather than critical care units for their basic pediatric rotation. Through a partnership with the University of Colorado School of Nursing, a Pediatric Critical Care course was developed in the summer of 2001. The course includes 3 days of classroom presentation and discussion and 60 hours of intensive, hands-on clinical experience in a higher acuity setting. These settings include the pediatric and newborn intensive care units and the emergency department. Junior- and senior-level students are encouraged to take this summer elective course if they wish to gain the critical-care clinical and assessment skills in pediatrics for the clinical assistant or graduate nurse role. Twelve students participated in the critical care course, six of whom were subsequently hired into the clinical assistant role.

STEP THREE: ACTIVE MENTORSHIP

Once new nurses have been hired, the hospital's responsibility continues in terms of education, mentorship, and support, so new staff feel connected to the hospital and to their particular units. This step of the process may be the most critical in retaining nurses who are qualified and satisfied in their work setting. Every newly hired RN participates in a centralized orientation program consisting of didactic learning and a precepted clinical experience. Those RNs hired as new graduates, those with little or no pediatric experience, and those reentering practice after extended time away are offered additional orientation through the Pediatric Nurse Development Program.

Four days of didactic instruction are provided for all new nurses, with 3 additional days for new graduates. On the additional days, topics range from pediatric fluid and electrolytes, chest tube management, and medication calculations, to facility information and scheduling opportunities. Additional unit-based classes follow centralized sessions and are tailored to meet the needs of the individual nurses and the specific pediatric population within departments. Evaluations from the Pediatric Nurse Development Program have been extremely positive. Nurses feel that the information covered is important and supplements what they received in school.

Continuing the professional development of nurses is a priority at TCH. Numerous hospital and community-based educational offerings are provided for mentoring clinically expert nurses, and scholarship funds are available to assist with tuition. Although the state of Colorado does not require continuing nursing education (CNE) for RN relicensure, TCH requires 10 contact hours annually. Staff can meet these requirements with the wide variety of internal CNE activities. Annual skills days provide hands-on methods to demonstrate competencies such as CPR, nursing roles in a respiratory or cardiac arrest, and managing chest tubes or central venous catheters. Unit-based "phase" classes were created to provide employees with didactic and hands-on unit-specific pediatric clinical skills. Examples of classes include oncologic emergencies, preparing for painful procedures, blood gas analysis, care of the pediatric spine-fusion patient, renal support systems, and "caring for yourself."

The Advanced Practice Nurses Council at TCH created a task force to examine how the nursing division can better mentor staff who are completing approximately 1 year of employment, but who are not yet seasoned nurses. The rationale to target this group of nurses is that once the formal orientation period is completed and staff are comfortable with the technical skills and tasks needed to function in their job, many are looking beyond the unit to identify other opportunities available for their own professional advancement. In our experience, between 1 and 2 years also is a critical time when the newly hired nurse is carefully evaluating the decision to stay in nursing as a career and at which specific institution. Thus, a group of advanced practice nurses volunteered to mentor these nurses and to serve as the liaison between the new employee and other TCH staff both within and across departments. Education coordinators, or nursing directors may also serve as mentors. Each mentor is encouraged to attend the TCH Mentorship workshop prior to serving in that function. This 3-hour workshop identifies differences between the preceptor and mentor role and describes characteristics of the novice-to-expert learner as characterized by Benner (2001). The role of the mentor is primarily to listen, support, and provide professional guidance as needed.

Protégés receive details of the program initially at hospital orientation and again at approximately 1-year post-hire from their managers. If interested, the name is forwarded to the mentorship task force where they are matched with a protégé. Mentors are encouraged to meet with their protégés, in a mutually agreed upon location, for approximately 1 hour monthly. Mentors and protégés keep a tracking log of their interactions, document their experiences, and make suggestions for areas needing improvement. The task force evaluates and makes necessary adjustments to the program. The goals of the mentorship program are for nurses to have a positive experience at TCH by enhancing their personal and professional growth and for the hospital to retain qualified staff.

In 1999, Mercer found that the underlying cause of staff turnover was dissatisfaction with the job, supervisor, or career prospects. Our own hospital Exit Evaluation Survey data showed staff nurse dissatisfaction with management. To address this concern, the Employee Opinion Survey and Manager Training Needs Assessment were conducted within the division of nursing.

In response to findings from these surveys, the Supervisory Management Certificate Program for Clinical Coordinators was created to augment the existing hospital-wide new-manager orientation. Clinical coordinators are frontline, unit-based managers, with authority to manage the unit staffing needs and to hire and discipline as needed. This program focuses on the basic skills needed to be an effective first-line supervisor. Case studies, open discussions, and simulations are used to explore and teach supervisory skills. Clinical coordinators must complete seven 4-hour core courses and one elective course in order to qualify for a certificate. Core courses include the following:

- Managing and Leading Your Employees
- Effective Communication and Listening Skills Training for Supervisors
- Performance Management and the Performance Review Process
- Customer Service Training for Supervisors
- Conflict Resolution and Negotiation Skills
- Decisionmaking and Problem Solving
- Team Building for Supervisors

Elective courses incorporate:

- Facilitating and Conducting Effective Meetings
- Effective Interviewing
- Motivating and Coaching Your Employees

STEP FOUR: TIME TO LISTEN

Retaining experienced, qualified nurses takes a concerted effort on the part of everyone in an organization. This effort begins with listening to staff and giving them a forum and a voice to be heard. It has been our experience that nurses who feel that they are listened to are more likely to remain in their jobs and serve as positive role models for others.

Comprised of staff nurses representing most programs within the division of nursing, a Clinical Nurse Council (CNC) was created to serve as a forum for communication between senior management, the executive team, and practicing staff. The group meets on a monthly basis and is facilitated by the vice president for patient care services. Institutional updates, issues of clinical relevance, as well as any other hot topics are discussed. Although there may not be resolution to a particular question or concern at the time, staff nurse members feel that they can make a difference in their clinical practice and that matters of importance to them are being acknowledged. Many times the nurses can resolve the issue, or come to an understanding, before the situation escalates.

The nursing Recruitment and Retention Committee, co-chaired by an inpatient-unit staff nurse and a nursing director, holds monthly meetings with all interested nurses from inpatient and outpatient areas to listen to and discuss ideas for recruitment and retention. The purpose of this committee is to share specific recruitment and retention feedback from staff and to make recommendations for changes to senior management. In 2001, group outcomes included support and direction for a revised hospital pension plan, weekend differential for difficult-to-fill positions, a new flexible scheduling program (9-month work year), enhanced staff recognition programs, and better communication between senior management and staff. This group is currently developing a nursing survey to identify workplace satisfiers.

In 2000, the Employee Opinion Survey was distributed to all employees. Senior management listened to staff concerns, resulting in an organizational action plan to focus on five key areas: pay, benefits, the performance appraisal system, communication, and staffing. Task forces were created and strategies were developed for addressing each specific area. Preliminary analysis of the same survey administered to employees in 2002 indicates a significant improvement perceived by staff in all domains.

SUMMARY

Although institutions cannot influence the increasing demand or the aging of current nursing staff, we can create programs to attract and retain competent nurses and future nursing leaders. The STAT four-step approach has demonstrated positive outcomes for our institution in several arenas:

• enhanced employee and student attraction to nursing careers through career days, cooperative education programs, elementary- and high-school visitations, and employee enrollment in nursing programs
• expanded employment opportunities for nursing students through the clinical technician and clinical assistant roles
• additional clinical education opportunities for students in critical care areas and pediatric classes for staff

TABLE 11.1 Nursing Hires at TCH 1999–2002

Year	No. of Hires
1999	87
2000	84
2001	110
2002	159

TABLE 11.2 Nursing Transfers Within TCH

Year	No. of Transfers
1999	39
2000	51
2001	65
2002	90

• greater number of nursing hires for 3 consecutive years (see Table 11.1)

• improved management, coaching, and supervising skills through the Clinical Coordinator Certificate program

• increased opportunities for professional growth through clinical precepting as a CTA, teaching as a CF, and mentoring newly hired staff

• better retention of staff through transfer within the TCH system (see Table 11.2).

No single factor contributed solely to these outcomes and the categories are neither mutually exclusive nor exhaustive. Rather, a combined effort within and across departments has led to the program's success. New strategies continue to be designed and implemented to attract and retain high-quality applicants into nursing.

REFERENCES

American Hospital Association, Strategic Policy Planning Committee. (2001, January). *Workforce supply for hospitals and health systems: Issues and recommendations.* Chicago, IL: Author.

Benner, P. E. (2001). *From novice to expert: Excellence and power in clinical nursing practice.* Upper Saddle River, NJ: Prentice-Hall.

Colorado State Board of Nursing, University of Colorado Health Sciences Center, and Colorado Area Higher Education Center. (2000). [Collaborative workforce data collection.] *Fact sheet: Registered Nurses in Colorado.* Denver, Colorado: Author.

Healthcare Information Resource Center. (1998). *1998 Nursing shortage study.* Walnut Creek, CA: Hay Group.

Hopkins, M. E. (2001). Critical condition. *NurseWeek (South Central), 6*(6), 21–24.

Joint Commission on Accreditation of Healthcare Organizations. (2002, August). *Health care at the crossroads: Strategies for addressing the evolving nursing crisis.* Retrieved December 4, 2002, from *http://www.jcaho.org/ news+room/news+release+archives/nursing+shortage.htm.*

Kimball, B., & O'Neil, E. (2002, April). *Health care's human crisis: The American nursing shortage.* Princeton, NJ: The Robert Wood Johnson Foundation.

Needleman, J., Buerhaus, P., Mattke, S., Stewart, M., & Zelevinsky, K. (2002). Nurse-staffing levels and the quality of care in hospitals. *New England Journal of Medicine, 346,* 1715–1722.

Peterson, C. A. (2001, January). Nursing shortage: Not a simple problem—no easy answers. *Online Journal of Issues in Nursing, 6*(1), 1. Retrieved January 31, 2001, from *http://www.nursingworld.org/ojin/topic14/tpc14_1.htm.*

U.S. Department of Health and Human Services, Health Resources and Services Administration, Bureau of Health Professions (2001, February). *The registered nurse population. National sample survey of registered nurses—March 2000. Preliminary findings.* Retrieved December 4, 2002, from *http:// purl.access.gpo.gov/GPO/LPS11936.*

U.S. Department of Health and Human Services, Health Resources and Services Administration, National Center for Health Workforce Analysis (2002, July). *Projected supply, demand, and shortages of registered nurses: 2000–2020.* Retrieved December 4, 2002, from *http://bhpr.hrsa.gov/healthworkforce/ rnproject/report.htm*

CHAPTER TWELVE

Responding to ANA's *Nursing's Agenda for the Future:* The Recruitment and Retention Program at a Major Medical Center

Christine Henriksen, Richard Williams II, Nancy E. Page, and Priscilla Sandford Worral

D espite the fact that nurses rank as "the nation's largest health care profession" (ANA, 2002, p. 5), the nation's health is critically threatened now and in the foreseeable future by a nursing shortage in our workforce. In mid 2001, the American Nurses Association (ANA) convened the Call to the Nursing Profession summit to take on three major tasks: to envision nursing's future, develop a strategic plan for attaining that future, and implement the plan. National nursing leaders who attended the summit accomplished the first two tasks, calling on the entire nursing community—indeed, the entire health care community—to take part in accomplishing the third.

Using *Nursing's Agenda for the Future* (ANA, 2002) and one of its 10 domains of focus as an organizing framework, this chapter describes how one institution, University Hospital, SUNY Upstate Medical University (Syracuse, New York), responded to the challenge of making nursing's vision for the future a reality. Within the recruitment and retention domain, nursing is envisioned as being "comprised of a diverse body of individuals committed to promoting and sustaining the profession through addressing diversity, image, education, funding,

practice models and environments, and professional development"
(ANA, p.17) where

- professional and career development opportunities are evident across the career span;
- funding is secured for creative educational initiatives that support nurses across the career span;
- nursing is seen as a highly desirable and appealing career choice;
- nurses develop professional practice models and work environments that ensure career satisfaction; and
- comprehensive recruitment and retention strategies demonstrate nursing's strong public image and appeal to a diverse population. (ANA, 2002, p. 17)

Because *Nursing's Agenda for the Future (Agenda)* is focused at the national level, the domain of recruitment and retention is similarly developed. The activities of recruitment and retention must take place at the local as well as national levels if they are to be successful. The strategies stated above are not mutually exclusive, but overlap one another, enabling organizational activities to address one or several strategies simultaneously. This chapter describes our institution's attempts to address recruitment and retention through creative initiatives, many of which are staff nurse driven. The *Agenda* calls for involvement of as many nurses as possible in charting their own future. Indeed, who could better recruit and retain staff nurses than staff nurses themselves? The *Agenda* was the ideal framework for use by our institution's chief nursing officer and chief operations officer. She holds a strong professional belief in the importance of a strategic plan to guide fiscally responsible allocation of scarce resources in an effort to empower staff to create a patient-focused, professionally nurturing environment.

STRATEGIES AND RELATED INITIATIVES: EDUCATION

Professional/career development opportunities are evident across the career span served as a primary strategy for identifying initiatives to be implemented or continued. Consistent with this central focus, *funding is secured for creative educational initiatives that support nurses across the career span* was selected as a secondary, more specific strategy. Initiatives driven by these strategies, described in some detail in the following sections, trace the career path of the professional nurse from pre-licensed student clinical assistant through specialty certified expert. In-service and continuing education activities are supported for nurses at all career stages to enable them to provide patient-focused, evidence-based nursing care.

STUDENT CLINICAL ASSISTANT PROGRAM

A valuable recruitment tool at our institution is the student clinical assistant (SCA) program, which allows nursing students to work as clinical assistants (unlicensed staff at the bedside) while still working on their nursing degree. This position entails providing direct patient care, including tasks such as phlebotomy, performing EKGs, and blood glucose monitoring. The SCA is not allowed to perform any tasks that fall within the scope of a licensed professional in New York State. Student nurses are mentored by staff RNs and work the same schedule as much as possible for continuity in the learning experience. Students are exposed to as many learning experiences as possible. For example, the SCA is permitted to observe a procedure such as chest tube insertion and assists the physician and RN while working within the restrictions of unlicensed personnel. This allows students to gain more clinical experience than is typical for an educational program. Students are usually in the junior year, or its equivalent, of their program. The hope of the supporting hospital is that the student nurse selects for employment the clinical unit where they were assigned as a student.

The SCA program has been a successful recruitment tool for our institution. The nursing recruitment department supports the salaries of the SCAs through their budget. Because SCAs are paid a straight hourly wage without benefits, they cost less to the institution than would a clinical assistant hired to accomplish the same work. The trends in hiring practices for this group are encouraging. In 1999, 51 SCAs were hired with 14 returning to be employed as graduate nurses (GNs). In 2000, 21 of 46 SCAs signed on as GNs and in 2001, 16 of 28 SCAs returned as GNs. This represents an almost 41% hiring rate. The 2-year retention rate for former SCAs who were hired in 2000 as GNs is 53%. Our 1-year retention rate for those SCAs hired in 2001 as GNs is 67%.

The SCA program does have similarities to graduate nurse intern programs across the country. In a study at Children's Hospital of Los Angeles, Beecroft, Kunzman, and Krozek (2001) found that nurse interns developed confidence, had the ability to provide competent care, and became committed to the organization. Certainly the rate of return experienced with the SCA program suggests that these nurses gained confidence while in the summer position and felt ready to commit later to the institution for employment.

NCLEX-RN Review Course

Providing opportunities for student nurses to be employed at the institution is the first step in recruitment and retention. Assisting the new graduate nurse to be successful on the NCLEX-RN is the next step in retention. The institution offers a class taught by two master's prepared nursing staff to prepare graduate nurses for the exam. These instructors are former or current nursing school instructors who update the course regularly so that it reflects the current trends in NCLEX-RN questions. Both instructors have developed and submitted questions for the exam and have published review texts.

The review course, covering clinical content and test-taking strategies, is viewed as having recruitment and retention functions. The course and review book are offered free of charge to all GNs employed at the facility. Nurses can attend class during the orientation period as part of their work schedule. The cost to the institution is estimated at $1,000 each time the course is offered, plus the salaries of the nurses attending. To date, 62 GNs have taken the hospital-based review course. The NCLEX-RN pass rate for graduate nurses taking this course was 97% in 2001 and 100% in 2002. Of the nurses who took the class in 2001, as many as 86% of those who passed were still employed in the hospital after 1 year. As of this writing, 88% of those who successfully took this course remain employed at our institution. In addition to NCLEX-RN preparation, this class offers the new graduate nurse an opportunity to have two mentors for support and encouragement during transition from senior nursing student to novice professional nurse. Further, GNs are encouraged to call either instructor with questions at any time.

Tuition Benefit Plans

Encouraging and financially supporting nurses to return to school for additional degrees is an effective retention tool. If an RN desires to return to school for advanced nursing education, he or she will be more likely to stay with the institution that is paying for the degree. RNs are required to be employed full time for 1 year to be eligible for tuition benefits from our institution. Because our facility is part of the state university system, we are able to provide tuition support equal to the state rate of $137 per credit hour for undergraduate courses and $237 per credit hour for graduate courses. Remitted tuition has also been available at a nearby private university as an agreement for precepting their undergraduate and graduate students. Unfortunately, this benefit will disappear over the next 4 years as the university closes its nursing program.

Collective bargaining units representing RNs also offer tuition reimbursement or professional study leaves to support further education. RNs may take advantage of these multiple sources of financial support to attend a more expensive program if they choose. Further education beyond the entry-level diploma, associate, or baccalaureate degree gives the RN higher-level analytic skills and often the confidence to pursue other opportunities in nursing, hopefully within the employing institution. Currently, 125 nursing and non-nursing staff are enrolled in multiple schools and colleges for various levels of nursing programs from basic to doctorate. Of the 720 RNs employed at the institution, 74 are currently enrolled in bachelor's or graduate programs.

Employers are challenged to make the work and professional environment attractive enough for RNs to remain and use their newfound skill sets in the institution where they started. We must be astute enough to grow RNs into administrative and clinical leadership roles while they work on the next degree. Assisting and advising RNs on clinical placements while in graduate school for nurse practitioner, clinical specialist, administration, and education roles can facilitate the employment of RNs in advanced positions with a demonstrated commitment to the institution.

In November 2002, our hospital agreed to a newly created position of academic advisor as part of federal health care worker retention dollars ($800,000) made available under the New York State Health Care Workforce Retention and Recruitment Act. It is the advisor's role to assist employees in determining what path to pursue, what education options are available, and what funding may be accessible. The advisor facilitates staff development to advance employee's careers in health care and at the same time retain those already employed at the institution.

FEDERAL GOVERNMENT LOAN REIMBURSEMENT

We began participating in the Nursing Education Loan Repayment Program (NELRP) from the Bureau of Health Professions of the U.S. Department of Health and Human Services (DHHS) in fall 2002 (DHHS, 2002). The federal government develops a list of eligible institutions in areas of nurse shortage, or those that fall into a particular type of institutional category. Facilities eligible to participate in NELRP include Indian Health Service Centers, Native Hawaiian Health Centers, public hospitals, migrant health centers, community health centers, health centers for the homeless, public-housing primary health centers, rural health clinics, and public or nonprofit private health facilities designated as having a critical shortage of RNs. Institutions that have applied and are considered eligible can be found on the Web site. Many facilities could not have budgeted for these loan repayment programs themselves.

Under this program, RNs prepared at all levels can have 85% of their nursing loans repaid by the federal government. The federal government, and not the institution, determines the applicant's eligibility. Employees must have a full-time contract at an eligible facility for at least 2 years. NELRP will pay 60% of the RN's total qualifying loan balance for 2 years of service or 85% for 3 years of service. Traveling or agency nurses are not considered eligible for this program. This works to the institution's benefit for recruitment and retention.

This program has resulted in an enormous boost to the recruitment and retention efforts for these institutions. Projected funding for NELRP for the year 2003 is $15 million, an increase of almost $4 million from the previous year and more than $13.8 million since 1999. Once an RN remains in an institution for 2 to 3 years to participate in the loan forgiveness program, it is anticipated that he or she will be more likely to stay on as a long-term employee.

SPECIALTY CERTIFICATION REIMBURSEMENT

We initiated a program to reimburse RNs for obtaining specialty certification and subsequent recertification. This is one of the many incentives that RNs have as they seek and continue employment. The hospital and its foundations also pay for most conferences and educational opportunities that the RN requires for contact hours needed to obtain and maintain certification. Evidence suggests that specialty certification is of benefit to the patient, the nurse, and the institution (Brady et al., 2001). Demonstrating the direct benefit of specialty certification to the professional presents a challenge because internal motivation and self-actualization are difficult to measure; however, evidence of such a benefit does exist (Carey, 2001).

Specialty certification has been associated with fewer health care errors (Carey, 2001). Nurses who are certified attribute the certification process itself as integral to improving their skills at detecting the clinical signs and symptoms of deterioration in the patients for whom they care (Carey). Some sources have termed this failure to detect impending shock and arrest as "failure to rescue" (Needleman, Buerhaus, Mattke, Stewart, & Zelevinsky, 2002). Research is ongoing to determine the effects of professional nursing certification on patient outcomes and the ability to prevent progression toward shock and subsequent cardiopulmonary arrest. Further, documenting the percentage of certified nurses is part of the application process for magnet-status credentialing through the American Nurses Credentialing Center (ANCC). Clearly, certification is considered a marker for excellence in nursing service and should be encouraged through institutional support.

Carey (2001) found that 72% of certified nurses surveyed realized rewards such as financial gain, promotions within the institution or their chosen specialty, job security, and recognition from colleagues and patients. These nurses also reported the benefit of increased confidence in their roles. Certification allowed the RN to grow professionally and experience greater satisfaction in the role of professional nurse. Carey also found that certified nurses gained new confidence in their profession and felt that they were viewed as credible providers. Recently we began to offer review courses for nurses who are preparing for certification exams. The cost to offer the review classes is $4,000–$4,500 per class, most of which is funded by a grant from our local professional nurses' union. Cost per class to the hospital is approximately $1,000.

Prior to summer 2002, the number of certified RNs employed was not tracked. In November 2002, however, the institution became an active member of the National Database for Nursing Quality Indicators in preparation for a magnet-status application. According to data then submitted on the acute care, acute medical surgical, and intensive care units at the hospital, 5.38% of staff RNs and 32% of nurse managers were certified. A process to maintain data on RNs who hold certification has been put into place, and we hope to see this number increase over time. Additionally, the chief nursing officer holds professional certification, a visible demonstration of her commitment to professional development.

CONTINUING EDUCATION

In addition to financially supporting nurses to hold specialty certification, numerous educational opportunities are offered. The Nursing Professional Development Council (NPDC), comprised primarily of staff nurses, coordinates a series of in-service programs for nursing staff. NPDC representatives use staff input to determine the content of these programs. Half-hour classes are offered consistently every 2 weeks, and nursing staff can schedule attendance at these sessions because they are always at the same time and place. NPDC is able to offer ANCC and state nursing association–approved contact hours for these programs through the university's Institute for Continuing Nursing Education. For each session, the nurse receives 0.6 contact hours.

Recently there has been a problem of low attendance at some sessions; nurses have voiced their frustration that staffing levels and workload make it difficult to attend. The NPDC has been working to make changes based on this feedback. NPDC has explored alternative activities, for example, that educational sessions are taped and made available on staff education television. Plans are in progress to have a traveling poster cart with a self-study guide and a posttest to enable nurses to access education on patient care units as time allows. We are investigating offering continuing education credits for these poster in-services.

Many other educational opportunities are available. Clinical nurse educators for core service lines offer classes pertinent to their specialty; these are open to nurses from other areas. For example, a nurse who works on a medical unit could review the training and development catalogue and sign up for a class offered by the critical care service line. Classes also are offered in computer skills, personnel management, and interpersonal skills. Opportunities can be tailored to the educational needs of participants

STRATEGIES AND RELATED INITIATIVES: SHARED GOVERNANCE

Nurses develop professional practice models and work environments that ensure career satisfaction was seen as a crucial secondary strategy that was consistent with the primary strategy of professional and career development opportunities. The transition of nursing from single department to institution-wide participant began even before *Nursing's Agenda for the Future* was written; it is likely to continue even as we near the "desired future state for nursing" (ANA, 2002, p. 6) in 2010.

Shared governance is important to an overall retention strategy. The new workers of today fully own the application of their skills. They are not likely to stay in a facility that does not value their contributions, or in one that assumes it owns both the workers and the work they perform (Porter O'Grady, 2001). Shared governance and point-of-care decision-making can be incorporated into the framework of an institution. According to Porter O'Grady shared governance is an ever changing and evolving process centered on four critical principles: partnership, accountability, equity, and ownership.

Shared governance has been defined as a model for empowering nurses and a framework for organizing nursing care (Howell et al., 2001). As an organization we developed a councilor structure of shared governance. Multiple councils exist within this structure, each with specific duties and functions. All councils have representatives from each core service within the hospital. The goal of utilizing this structure is to involve as many RNs as possible in making decisions that affect their practice, education, and management.

The Nursing Coordinating Council (NCC) provides oversight for the councils, establishing operation guidelines and facilitating cross-council communication and oversight of the nursing quality indicator report for the institution. The coordinator for nursing practice and the chief nursing officer cochair the NCC. Members include the cochairs of the other councils, nurse researcher, nurse epidemiologist, and dean of the college of nursing.

The Nursing Operations Council (NOC), cochaired by two nursing directors and comprised of the nurse administrators and patient service managers, is responsible for daily nursing operations issues and for reviewing and monitoring the utilization of nursing resources. The Nursing Practice Council (NPC), cochaired by staff RNs and comprised of direct care nurses from each service line, is responsible for creating and revising clinical policies, incorporating standards of nursing into policy and practice, and reviewing nursing quality cases. The NPDC, cochaired by a staff nurse and nurse clinical educator and comprised of direct care nurses from each service line, facilitates staff nurse pursuit of national specialty certification and offers individual self-directed learning to accomplish that goal. NPDC developed and maintains a clinical orientation pathway for new GNs and recognizes preceptors for their role in training and retaining nurses.

The Nursing Research Council (NRC) is cochaired by staff nurses, coached by the coordinator for nursing research, and comprised of direct care nurses from each service line, a nurse member of the hospital ethics committee, and a nurse case manager. Ad hoc members include a librarian, the nurse epidemiologist, and the dean of the college of nursing. The NRC facilitates evidence-based practice by searching for, reviewing, and critiquing evidence relevant to issues identified by direct care nurses. The NRC also assists the NPC in establishing evidence-based policies. The Recruitment, Retention and Recognition Advisory Group (3R), cochaired by staff nurses, is primarily responsible for strategies to retain professional nursing staff and recognize all levels of nursing staff. The councilor structure also includes an ambulatory care council, again comprised of professional nursing staff, to address the practice and operations issues relevant to their patients and the ambulatory care environment. Figure 12.1 shows a model of a nursing council structure.

How has this model of shared governance impacted on the retention of professional nurses? By bringing staff nurses into decision-making roles, they become empowered. Because the governance

Nursing Council Structure

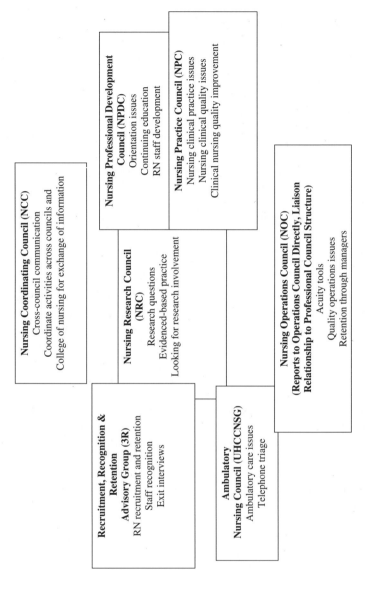

FIGURE 12.1 Nursing Council Structure.

structure involves nursing staff in day-to-day decision-making they are more likely to remain employed in this facility. Over the last 5 years, a majority of staff who have been retained had been active on councils. The retention rate is even greater for staff that held leadership roles on the councils; 100% of staff that held a chair position on a council remain employed at the institution.

IMPACT OF THE SHARED GOVERNANCE STRUCTURE

Prior to developing the council structure, administrators and managers made the majority of decisions regarding professional practice, with little or no input from bedside nurses. Directors led most hospital committees. Even if staff nurses served on committees, they felt they had little input in decision making. It was early in 1996 that the concept of shared governance was implemented. From the outset, with the initiation of this model, nurses began to see tangible changes. Staff nurses began to make decisions that directly affected nursing practice. Staff RNs soon replaced managers and administrators in leading committees that directly affected patient care, staff recruitment, and professional nursing education. Within a year, staff nurses were not only part of the decision-making process, they were leading councils and committees and participating in change. The power base for decisions affecting the bedside nurse shifted to the nurses themselves.

The greatest impact has been seen during the orientation of new nurses. In 1999, the NPDC surveyed RNs with less than 2 years of experience. Over 60% of respondents stated that they did not feel comfortable working alone when their orientation was completed. Staff nurses on this council decided to evaluate how new staff were oriented. What we found was surprising. Orientation of new nurses ranged from 6 to 16 weeks. Those areas that had a comprehensive 16-week orientation experienced better retention of new GNs. The NPDC saw this as an opportunity for sweeping change. After seeking input from their respective service lines, NPDC members devised a standardized, comprehensive orientation plan that could be adapted to the new GN's comfort level. A 16-week plan was developed with the opportunity for adaptation to the comfort and skill of the new graduate. Intended to foster teamwork and a professionally nurturing environment as well as improve technical skill, the plan focuses on the basics of nursing as well as team building, and it gradually progresses to independently caring for a diverse patient population. During the orientation, RNs are given specific time to work with all of the health team members.

Since the plan was initiated in late spring 2000, NPDC members have collected data to evaluate the use and effectiveness of this revised orientation process. With the assistance of the Nursing Research Council, data collection was completed and results will be available in 2003. Initial results of data analysis show a slight increase in satisfaction of RN staff. Pending further evaluation, NPDC members will work on making additional changes in the orientation of new RNs.

GROWTH OF SHARED GOVERNANCE

Shared governance continues to grow and evolve. Challenges remain, however, for example, how to maximize the involvement of the remaining professional nursing staff in this participatory model of governance. As with any change, resistance can be an issue. Those clinical areas with staff nurses chairing one of the councils have demonstrated a better understanding of the councilor model of shared governance. Numerous modes of communication are used to market the councils' activities across units and shifts. Each council representative is responsible for bringing information from the council to her or his respective service line to solicit feedback. The flow of communication allows for each professional nurse's voice to be heard, yet not all nurses take advantage of this opportunity. New nursing staff members are encouraged to attend a council meeting during their orientation to learn more about the governance structure. By supporting this model of shared governance, nurses have the opportunity to shape the environment where they practice, control the direction of their own professional development, and plan the strategies that support staff recruitment and retention.

The next step is to take RN autonomy to the unit level. Allowing staff to have a voice in the day-to-day decision making on nursing units, including budgetary decisions, staffing patterns, and scheduling, can maximize autonomy. The value of unit-level decisions and the role these decisions play in operationalizing RN autonomy still needs to be defined in the current model of shared governance.

A shared governance structure should never remain static. As with any change, a period of reevaluation and restructuring is needed to evaluate outcomes and make further changes. Further, although shared governance has spread to the staff nurse leader, there is a need to assess whether or not the structure is effective in reaching nurses who are working at the bedside.

SUMMARY

Among the efforts described in the literature are those that serve to recruit and to retain registered professional nurses. Often what attracts the RN to an employer is identical to that which retains the RN over the long term. It is well known that key to maintaining a stable workforce is creating an environment where the employee wants to stay (Joint Commission on the Accreditation of Health Care Organizations [JCAHO], 2002). This situation is not unique to hospitals. Any business, public or private, for profit or not for profit, thrives when their workforce is experienced and empowered. Our institution is dedicated to creating an environment that nurtures the development and autonomy of the professional nurse.

Our commitment to nursing is demonstrated through providing employment opportunities for student nurses, tuition support and tuition reimbursement, and professional certification and recertification reimbursement, and by offering continuing education opportunities in various venues and encouraging the involvement of all professional nurses in the shared governance structure. The professional needs of nurses change over the span of their careers. Employers must offer a wide variety of services to address the changing needs of nurses in order to retain dedicated professionals. Using strategies identified in *Nursing's Agenda for the Future* as a guide to recruitment and retention serves us well because they assist us in meeting our obligation not only to nurses in our institution, but to the nursing profession and to the community we serve.

REFERENCES

American Nurses Association (2002). Nursing's agenda for the future. Washington, DC: American Nurses Publishing.

Beecroft, P., Kunzman, L., & Krozek, C. (2001), RN internship: Outcomes of a one-year pilot program. *Journal of Nursing Administration, 31,* 575–582.

Brady, C., Becker, K., Brigham, L., Goldman, J., Wilson, B., & George, E. (2001). The case for mandatory certification. *Journal of Nursing Administration, 31,* 466–467.

Carey, A. (2001). Certified registered nurses: Results of the study of the certified workforce. *American Journal of Nursing, 101,* 44–52.

Clipp, E. C. (2001). Can nurses govern in a government agency? *Journal of Nursing Administration, 31,* 187–195.

Joint Commission on the Accreditation of Healthcare Organizations (2002). News from the JOAHO. Health care at the crossroads: Strategies for addressing the evolving nursing crisis. *Journal of Clinical Systems Management, 4*(10), 9, 18.

Needleman, J., Buerhaus, P., Mattke, S., Stewart, M., & Zelevinsky, K. (2002). Nurse-staffing levels and the quality of care in hospitals. *New England Journal of Medicine, 346,* 1715–1722.

Porter O'Grady, T. (2001). Is shared governance still relevant? *Journal of Nursing Administration, 31,* 468–473.

U.S. Department of Health and Human Services. Nursing Education Loan Repayment Program. Retrieved July 8, 2002, from *http://bhpr.hrsa.gov/nursing/loanrepay.htm.*

CHAPTER THIRTEEN

Career Development Programs at an Icelandic Hospital

Hrafn Óli Sigurðsson

A s the shortage of nurses is felt in hospitals around the globe, the recruitment and retention of nurses have become more important than ever. A major contributing factor to the shortage is fewer enrollments in nursing programs, resulting in fewer nurses entering the workforce. With a smaller number of new and younger nurses, the current nursing population is aging faster than other workforce groups, with the potential for an even greater shortage as these older nurses retire (Staiger, Auerbach, & Buerhaus, 2000). Another aspect of the shrinking nursing workforce is attrition, as demonstrated in a survey among newly graduated nurses in England, where one in four did not expect to be working in nursing in 5 years (Parish, 2002).

When faced with a limited number of nurses, nursing administrators must actively implement retention programs. Although there is no quick fix to reduce staff turnover since it is influenced by the organizational culture (Contino, 2002), one approach to retain nurses is to offer programs that assist them in developing their careers ("Getting and keeping the best and the brightest," 2000). Increased knowledge and competence is of mutual interest to both individual nurses and their employers, and the desire among nurses for increased challenges and career development opportunities through continued educational activities is common (Urden, 1999). This chapter describes the approach taken at Landspítali University Hospital in Reykjavik, Iceland, to conceptualize and begin implementation of a comprehensive career development strategy in an effort to attract and retain nurses.

BACKGROUND OF LANDSPÍTALI UNIVERSITY HOSPITAL

The Icelandic Nurses Association recently estimated the national nursing shortage in Iceland to be 14% based on all budgeted registered
nurse positions. This number has been similar in surveys conducted
previously (Félag íslenskra hjúkrunarfræðinga, 1999). The vacancy rate
at the Landspítali University Hospital, the biggest single employer of
nurses in Iceland, has been around 10%. Landspítali University Hospital (LUH) was created in May 2000 from the merger of two major
hospitals in Reykjavik, Iceland. With the creation of a new 995-bed
hospital we needed to rethink the organization of nursing services.
One of the pre-merger hospitals had for several years a successful
internship program for new graduates consisting of clinical rotations
in two units, formal educational days, and group supervision. The
challenge was to use that experience to restructure and expand career development opportunities for nurses in the new combined institution.

In an effort to evaluate the existing internship program for new
nurses and to formulate a new approach to orientation, an ad hoc task
force of five nurses, including three staff nurses, one educator, and
one administrator, was created in late 2000. The task force was given
2 months to present its recommendations. Three focus groups were
held to collect data from the hospital staff, and an e-mail survey was
conducted with the graduating nursing class during a period of 2 weeks
in early January 2001 (Sigurdsson, Bragadottir, Gudmundsdottir, Magnusson, & Sigurjonsdottir, 2001). This article summarizes each element in the process of data collection and describes achieved and
proposed outcomes.

DATA COLLECTION AND EVALUATION

The three focus groups consisted of newly graduated nurses, experienced nurses, and nurse managers, respectively. The purposes of the
focus groups were to elicit perceptions about existing programs and
invite suggestions for improvement. The focus groups were held in a
hospital meeting room during work hours and refreshments were
served as a token of appreciation. Two members of the Task Force
facilitated each focus group and alternated in that responsibility. Typical questions posed to the groups were: What is important to new
graduates as they enter their first job? What is your experience and
opinion of the existing internship program? What type of support is
needed for new graduates? Is one type of program enough for the

institution? Each session lasted about 1 hour, during which detailed written notes were taken by one of the facilitators outlining the discussion points. Additionally, each session was tape recorded as a backup for clarification purposes. The recording facilitator prepared a written thematic summary of each group by reviewing the notes taken during each session. The summary was considered accurate if both facilitators agreed on its content.

FOCUS GROUP RESULTS

The first group consisted of seven nurses who were in their second year of practice. Group members indicated that those who participated in the internship program were pleased with the experience and recommended that all new graduates be encouraged to participate. They felt that the internship should offer clinical experience in general medical/surgical units and that specialized units, such as the ICU or ER, should be reserved for another level or program. These nurses emphasized the benefit and support of the supervision groups as an integral part of the internship program. They also talked about the importance of an active in-service education program, both for the internship program and also for nurses in general. They felt that the availability of a resource person, for example, a nurse educator or a clinical specialist, would provide the nursing staff with much needed educational support and encouragement for research.

The second focus group was comprised of 6 nurses with 5 or more years of experience. They felt that the previous internship program had given good results and had been well liked by the participants they knew. They felt the internship program should be continued, but that participation should be optional for new graduates, especially if they wished to spend the entire 12 months on one unit. A specialized internship program was seen as a positive option for nurses to expand and simultaneously focus their clinical experience in a specific area. They felt, however, that as had been experienced occasionally in the past, nurse managers might be reluctant to support a program that could encourage nurses to move on from their units. They liked the idea of cross training but foresaw implementation difficulties except where there was optimal staffing in all areas involved. They feared that some services might be more popular, attracting more staff, which would not be fair to other services. The experienced nurses recommended that points, or continuing education credits, be given for attending educational activities to increase attendance. They supported the idea of educators who would serve as liaisons to the Faculty of Nursing at the University of Iceland. They similarly emphasized the importance of unit-based orientation and organized educational material specific to each unit.

Eight nurse managers and preceptors attended the third focus group. This group felt that a minimal stay on a unit should be a 6-month period during the internship. They felt that most new graduates were "thirsty" for work and thus it was unrealistic to expect much reading or studying during the first few months. New graduates, in their experience, often take their first position on a unit where they have had a good student rotation, which highlights the importance that all staff members be motivated to give students a supportive and varied experience. Along this line of thought they recommended that a designated person be assigned to new orientees on each unit, although they also recognized that in reality that often proved difficult because of staffing issues. They had observed that often after about 2 years new staff would become eager for new challenges that managers and preceptors had little flexibility to provide. They noted that group supervision during the internship program was generally well liked by the new nurses and recommended that supervision be more readily available to all staff. They also stated that educational activities during the internship program must not be a repeat of material graduates have already had during their senior year, as sometimes seems to be the case.

E-mail Survey

A short questionnaire was prepared which was intended to elicit the expectations of students in the graduating nursing class. The questionnaire consisted of nine items; six of these were open-ended questions asking the respondents to identify what factors were most influential in choosing an employer and if they had already decided where they would work after graduation. The remaining three items listed workplace characteristics that the respondents were asked to rank according to perceived importance.

In 1986 entry into professional nursing practice in Iceland was established as being exclusively via a 4-year baccalaureate nursing education at either the University of Iceland in Reykjavik or University of Akureyri in northern Iceland. In 2001, the graduating class consisted of 84 students from the two universities, which is a good number since only 90 students are allowed to proceed after their first semester of study due to limitations set by the nursing programs. Both nursing programs were contacted to obtain a list of graduating students' e-mail addressees. The survey was sent once in early January to all 84 students and yielded 27 responses, or 32%. The students were instructed to use the "reply with history" option and enter their responses to the questions directly into the document. Responses were printed and names cut off to maintain responder anonymity; simple frequencies were then tallied. Each e-mail response was deleted immediately after printing.

E-MAIL SURVEY RESULTS

When asked what the dominant factor is when deciding where to work, 74% mentioned good salary, 48% mentioned an interesting/exciting and challenging job, 41% mentioned good coworkers, and 40%, a reasonable workload. Most (70%) had not decided in January where they intended to work by graduation in June. During orientation, enough time to feel confident was most important to 52% of the respondents. Good unit organization and standardized procedure manuals were mentioned by 41%. Another 33% wished for an experienced RN preceptor.

Projecting ahead 5 years, 59% of these nursing students hoped to be very competent nurses. Thirty-seven percent said they hoped to have completed additional or graduate education in 5 years. Positive work morale, support, and encouragement by peers were considered important by 44% to best realize this goal, together with their own commitment, interest, and hard work (33%). The most prevalent expectations toward their prospective employer were clearly centered on professional growth, increased knowledge and competence, and good compensation (See Table 13.1).

Working hours for nurses in Iceland have traditionally been rotating 8-hour shifts, covering days (D), evenings (E), and nights (N). Only in rare instances are permanent shifts assigned. Recently, other possibilities have been implemented and the nursing students who participated indicated that they wished to work every third weekend (44%), only two out of three shifts (mostly D/E, D/N) (26%), or to create their own schedule (22%). When asked to rank the most important expecta-

TABLE 13.1 Selected Workplace Expectations of Nursing Students Completing Baccalaureate-Nursing Education (N = 27)

- Interesting/challenging work (85%)[a]
- Good salary (81%)
- Professional group supervision (44%)
- Working the same shifts as the preceptor (40%)
- Onsite clinical specialization courses/training (37%)
- Onsite graduate courses (26%)

[a]Values represent percentages of responses.

tions about their work environment, 59% wanted upbeat and good coworkers, 37% felt computer access was important, 26% ranked a unit-based staff lounge for meals and breaks as important, and 22% mentioned onsite child day care.

RETENTION STRATEGIES

Successful recruitment and retention depend on a clear and comprehensive policy on what orientation and career development opportunities the institution offers ("Getting and keeping . . ." 2000). Options must be available to nurses throughout their careers that support and encourage professional development in response to their desire for increased competence (Urden, 1999). Successful retention strategies should take into account the needs and wishes of the next generation of professionals who expect balanced lives, personal and professional growth, rewards for accomplishments, and a sense of community at work (Hill & Ingala, 2002; Izzo & Withers, 2002).

Results of the focus group of nurses in their second year of practice and the survey of the graduating class emphasized orientation and support of interesting work where they have control over their working hours and schedule. This is consistent with typical expectations of members of so-called Generation X, who stay in a job only as long as it is interesting, they can learn new things and grow, and they can "have a life" of their own through a flexible work schedule (Cordeniz, 2002). In order to reduce turnover, these expectations need to be addressed by creating a culture that is attentive and fosters two-way communication between nursing staff and managers (Contino, 2002).

RECOMMENDATIONS

The desire for professional development to maintain and improve competence was clearly evident in the focus groups as well as students in the graduating class. The committee quickly identified that although a successful internship program had been an option for new graduates for years, in order to foster retention a different, more comprehensive approach for both new graduates and incumbent RNs was needed.

A THREE-LEVEL CAREER DEVELOPMENT STRATEGY

After careful analysis of data from the focus groups and the e-mail survey, the task force proposed a new three-level career development structure that would be responsive to the needs for advancement and increased professional competence. The first level is a General Internship Program. The second level is a Specialty Internship Program, and the third level is a Service-Focused Cross Training Program. These programs were designed to assist nurses individually in professional growth and also, from an organizational point of view, to facilitate the development of competent, knowledgeable staff. A summary of each program follows.

General Internship Program. This program is designed for the new graduate. The program is 12 months in duration starting September 15 each year and consists of three components: clinical rotations, supervision, and education. Based on each applicant's interests identified in an individual interview about 3 to 4 months before graduation, rotations of various clinical experiences are planned. New graduates can choose to stay for the entire 12-month period in one clinical area or divide the time between two or three areas to begin to achieve their professional goals.

Supervision is done bi-weekly in 1.5-hour sessions from September through May in small groups of six to eight. The principles of clinical supervision of predetermined regular meeting time, committed attendance and confidentiality are observed in these meetings. The groups are lead by experienced supervisors who do not serve in any other capacity to the nurses. This is done so that the new graduates feel free to express whatever issues they may have in the group in confidence, without fear of any management repercussions. Issues are taken outside the group with the group's permission if they need administrative resolution.

The educational component is achieved during 5 full-day workshops from October through April, focusing on clinical, safety, professional, and organizational issues. It was decided that full-day programs would be the easiest for staff scheduling as opposed to half-day programs. These days are considered work on the day shift. Instructional methods include lecture, discussion, case studies, and site visits.

Specialty Internship Program. As a second level for career development, the committee proposed a new internship program open to nurses who had completed the General Internship Program or who had at least 1 year of work experience. Because of a shortage of specialized nurses at the hospital, this pilot program was proposed for perioperative, anesthesia, and critical care areas. An important component of this program is collaboration between the University Hospital and the Faculty of Nursing at the University of Iceland. The University provides the theory part of the program for academic credit, which can be applied toward a master's degree. The University Hospital provides the clinical experiences.

Guidelines from the European Union about professional education transferability as well as any international or professional standards set by each specialty organization provide the minimum standards for the design of this program. Upon completing the 30-credit, 18-month program, students will receive a diploma in Specialized Nursing from the Faculty of Nursing. This is seen as a prototype program that can be applied to many other nursing specialties. Negotiations are underway between the University Hospital and the Faculty of Nursing to move this recommendation to action, with a start date of fall 2003. More details will be published as the program is implemented and subsequently evaluated.

Service Focused Cross Training Program. This program is conceptualized for nurses with at least 2 years of experience who want to expand their expertise to another unit. The new approach to traditional cross training is to focus on certain patient populations in the different units and settings where they receive care (Sigurdsson, 2000). For example, a nurse interested in cardiology patients might choose to expand his or her training to care for those patients in the outpatient, inpatient, and critical care settings. Another example might be a nurse interested in ENT patients who decides to acquire skills to work with these patients in the OR, inpatient, or outpatient clinic setting.

The cross training program is based on nurses' clinical interests in becoming more skilled and experienced within a certain patient population rather than as a response to the institution's need for flexible staff. With this focus nurses are in charge of their clinical development and more cohesiveness across different units is anticipated. Similar to the General Internship program, an educational component as well as group supervision are planned to be an integral part of this program. This proposal has been well received and several nurses have expressed interest, although at the time of this writing an implementation date has yet to be determined.

PROGRAM EVALUATION

In the first year of operation, the General Internship program had 31 participants. An anonymous mailed evaluation upon completion of the program yielded 22 (71%) responses, 18 completed surveys and 4 incomplete surveys from nurses no longer employed at the hospital. Of the 31 initial participants 24 (77%) were still employed at the end of the 12-month program, and seven (23%) had left, as indicated by payroll department data. Based on the four responses from the nurses who left, two gave low pay as a reason for leaving and two had moved abroad. It is difficult to evaluate the attrition of 23% since no prior data exist from before the merger regarding attrition; however, trends will be monitored closely as the General Internship Program continues. At the time of this writing the second group is in the middle of their program and applicants for the third group are being interviewed. A study among nurses who have left LUH during the period of 2000 to 2002 is currently in progress; results from this study, together with continued evaluation of the Internship Programs, are expected to provide valuable information for future adjustments and policy development.

The evaluation questionnaire consisted of 71 items, 36 relating to the clinical settings and satisfaction, 13 relating to the educational portion, 10 relating to the supervision, and the remaining 12 items eliciting general satisfaction with the program and perceptions about career development opportunities at the hospital. Space was provided in each section for additional written comments.

With regard to program satisfaction, responses were generally positive and provide encouragement for further refinement of the career development programs (see Table 13.2). Areas for improvement are

TABLE 13.2 Evaluation of General Internship Program (N = 18)[b]

Representative statements	Agree or Strongly agree[a]	Mean[b]	Standard Deviation
The period on this unit met my expectations	94	3.67	.59
The unit orientation met my needs	78	3.41	.79
I had a designated preceptor	61	2.94	1.30
I worked with competent RNs	100	3.78	.42
The manager was supportive	83	3.22	.73
The number of educational days was adequate (5 days)	94	3.59	.51
The group supervision helped me adjust to a new role	89	3.41	.62
The group supervision is an important part of the Internship Program	94	3.88	.33
The Internship Program design is as it should be	83	2.88	.33
I intend to enroll in the Specialty Internship Program	67	2.80	.68
I intend to enroll in the Service Focused Cross Training Program	33	2.27	.88
I am happy with my Internship Program	100	3.28	.46
I see good opportunities for career advancement at the hospital	78	3.00	.79

[a]Values represent percentages of responses.

[b]Likert scale where 1 = Strongly Disagree, 2 = Disagree, 3 = Agree, 4 = Strongly Agree.

that nursing units should be encouraged to develop their unit-specific orientation plans and ensure that each orientee has a designated preceptor. A few written comments in the evaluation referred to some repetition of material during the educational days that had been covered during the senior year in nursing school. This will be addressed through periodic review of course descriptions and lecture topics.

Participants indicated an interest in the other two proposed career development programs, especially the Specialty Internship Program (67%). Although interest in the Service-Focused Cross Training Program (33%) is moderate, the data are encouraging as this is a new approach to developing one's nursing career. Other suggestions from the focus groups are being considered. A job description for the clinical nurse specialist (CNS) role has been completed, although CNS job lines have not been created at the time of this writing. The LUH educational division has expressed interest in looking into awarding contact hours for educational activity.

CONCLUSION

There is a great need to recruit and retain nurses in all health care settings. An important strategy in retention is to offer education and career development options that are readily available (Kramer & Schmalenberg, 2002). Based on data from the focus groups of practicing nurses, managers and preceptors and an e-mail survey of students in the graduating nursing class, a new structure for career development consisting of a three-level program was proposed. This approach is ambitious; however, despite the usual skepticism associated with implementation of a new initiative, the ideas have been well received among nurses and managers. Progress is evident and new graduates have quickly shown their satisfaction with the revised General Internship Program. As the other two levels of the career development structure are implemented, careful tracking of the effectiveness of all three levels as recruitment and retention strategies, as well as ongoing evaluation of staff satisfaction with the programs, will be needed.

REFERENCES

Contino, D. S. (2002). How to slash costly turnover. *Nursing Management, 33*(2), 10–13.

Cordeniz, J. A. (2002). Recruitment, retention, and management of Generation X: A focus on nursing professionals. *Journal of Healthcare Management, 47*(4), 237–249.

Félag íslenskra hjúkrunarfræðinga. (1999, March). *Mannekla í hjúkrun* [The nursing shortage]. Reykjavik, Iceland: Author.

Getting and keeping the best and the brightest: An AONE executive summary. (2000). *Nursing Management, 31*(5), 17.

Hill, K., & Ingala, J. (2002). Just ask them! *Nursing Management, 33*(10), 21–22.

Izzo, J. B., & Withers, P. (2002). Winning employee-retention strategies for today's healthcare organizations. *Helathcare Financial Management, 56*(6), 52–57.

Kramer, M., & Schmalenberg, C. (2002). Staff nurses identify essentials of magnetism. In M. L. McClure & A. S. Hinshaw (Eds.), *Magnet hospitals revisited: Attraction and retention of professional nurses* (pp. 25–59). Washington, DC: American Nurses Association.

Parish, C. (2002). One in four new staff plan to quit within five years. *Nursing Standard, 16*(42), 5.

Sigurdsson, H. O. (2000, August). *Líkan fyrir hjúkrun í sérgreinum* [Model for specialty nursing delivery]. Reykjavik, Iceland: Landspitali University Hospital: Nursing Development Office.

Sigurdsson, H. O., Bragadottir, G., Gudmundsdottir, H. Y., Magnusson, C., & Sigurjonsdottir, Þ. I. (2001, January). *Skýrsla nefndar um móttöku og aðlögun nýrra hjúkrunarfræðinga* [Committee report on reception and orientation of new nurses]. Reykjavik, Iceland: Landspítali University Hospital, Nursing Development Office.

Staiger, D. O., Auerbach, D. I., & Buerhaus, P. I. (2000). Expanding career opportunities for women and the declining interest in nursing as a career. *Nursing Economics, 18*(5), 230–236.

Urden, L. D. (1999). What makes nurses stay? *Nursing Management, 30*(5), 27, 30.

Major Reports on the Nursing Shortage

American Association of Colleges of Nursing. (1999). Order No. 99-0185(P). Washington, DC: Author.

American Organization of Nurse Executives. (2000). Perspectives on the nursing shortage: A blueprint for action. Washington, DC. 73 pp. Online: *http://www.aone.org.*

American Organization of Nurse Executives. *Nurse recruitment and retention study.* Chicago, IL: AONE Institute for Patient Care Research and Education, 2000. Online: *http://www.aone.org.*

Bednash, G. (2000, June 14). The decreasing supply of registered nurses. Inevitable future or call to action? *JAMA, 283*(22), 2985–2987.

Buerhaus, P. I., Staiger, D. O., & Auerbach, D. I. (2000). Implications of an aging registered nurse workforce. *JAMA, 283,* 2948–2954.

Faso, J. J., O'Connell, M., & Hays, J. (2001). *Resolving New York's nursing shortage: Recommendations for addressing the nursing shortage in New York State.* A Report from The Assembly Minority Nursing Shortage Task Force. 34 pp.

GNYHA (2001, April 19). Survey of nurse staffing in hospitals in the New York City Region 2001. Greater New York Hospital Association, New York, NY. 24 pp.

HANYS. (2000, December). *The crisis in care: Health care workforce shortages.* Healthcare Association of New York State, New York, NY. Online: *http://hanys.org.*

JCAHO. (2002, August). *Health care at the crossroads: Strategies for addressing the evolving nursing crisis.* Joint Commission on Accreditation of Healthcare Organizations. 43 pp. Online: *http://www.jcaho.org.*

Kimball, B., & O'Neil, E. O. (2002, April). *Health care's human crisis: The American nursing shortage.* Report of the Robert Wood Johnson Foundation. The Robert Wood Johnson Foundation, Princeton, NJ. 82 pp. Online: *http://www.rwjf.org.*

Mailey, S. S., Charles, J., Piper, S., Hunt-McCool, J., Wilborne-Davis, P., & Baigis, J. (2000). Analysis of the nursing work force compared with national trends. *Journal of Nursing Administration, 30*(10), 482–489.

Martin, L. (2001, May). *Who will care for each of us? American's coming health care labor crisis.* A Report from the Panel on The Future of the Health Care Labor Force in a Graying Society. University of Illinois at Chicago College of Nursing, Nursing Institute. Chicago, IL. 33 pp. Online: *http://www.uluc.edu/nursing/nursinginstitute.*

New York State Education Department Office of the Professions. (2001, June 21). The Nursing Shortage. Report to the New York State Board of Regents. Albany, NY: Author. 17 pp., Online: *http://www.op.nysed.gov/nurse shortage.htm.*

Perez, A. (2002, June). *Closing the nursing gap.* Report of The City University of New York Nursing Task Force. New York, NY. 8 pp.

Smith, J., & Crawford, L. (2002, May 9). *Findings from the 2001 employers survey.* National Council of State Boards of Nursing. NCSBN Research Brief, Volume 3 (2002). Online: *http://www.ncsbn.org/public/resources/resources_publication.htm.*

USDHHS (2002, July). *Projected supply, demand, and shortages of registered nurses: 2000–2020.* Washington, DC: 22 pp. U.S. Department of Health and Human Services, Health Resources and Services Administration Bureau of Health Professions, National Center for Health Workforce Analysis.

Williams, C. A. (2001). The RN shortage: Not just nursing's problem. *Academic Medicine, 76*(3), 218–220.

Index

Perception of profession, 10, 11
Personal qualities, new graduates,
    97–100
Pool of qualified nursing faculty,
    shrinking of, 3
Power sharing, nurse retention and,
    120–135
  challenge, 123
  control, 124
  discipline, 124
  leadership, 124–125
  meetings, 129–130
  nurse executives, 131–132
  nursing satisfaction, 125–126
  openness, 123
  organizational characteristics,
      empowerment and, 123–124
  personal characteristics, 131
  power
    dimensions of, 121–123
    understanding, 120–123
  security, 124
  strategies, 128–131
  support, 124
  teamwork, 123
  transfer of power, across
      organization, 125–126
  transformational leaders, 127–128
  vision, 123
Professional group supervision, 167
Professional qualities, of new
    graduates, 97–100
Public relations, operating room
    nurse shortage and, 49–50

Recruitment, Recognition and
    Retention Advisory Group,
    158
Registered Nurse Relicensure
    Survey, likeliness to leave
    primary position, 15
Repayment program, loan, Vermont,
    nursing education, 17
Research, classes in, in Kennesaw
    State University School of
    Nursing curriculum, 75

Retention strategies, 168
Rotations, clinical, in STAT!
    Program, instructors to
    supervise students in, 142
Rural state nursing shortage,
    Nevada, 34–44
  evaluation, 43
  higher education in Nevada, 36
  Hospital Association, statewide
      task force, 34–43
  transformational nursing
      leadership theory, 35

Salaries, nursing, increase in, 20
Scholarship support, from private
    sources, for nursing
    students, 17–18
Schools, nursing, role of, 57–69
  competency
    in leadership, 65
    in management, 65
  Council on Collegiate Education
      for Nursing, 57
  diversity, increasing, 61–62
  faculty shortages, dealing with, 66–67
  financial barriers to education,
      reducing, 62–63
  government, advocacy, 63
  image of nursing, enhancing, 60
  interdisciplinary education, for
      collaborative practice, 65–66
  international solutions, 63–64
  strategic partnerships, 59
  technology, 64–65
  youth awareness, 60–61
Semester, Kennesaw State
    University School of Nursing
    curriculum, 75
Senior baccalaureate nursing
    students, success in
    workplace, perceptions of,
    94–104
  intraprofessional alliances, 98, 102
  organizational culture, 97–98, 100
  personal qualities, new graduates,
    97–100

Springer Publishing Company

— Journal —

Nursing Leadership Forum

Harriet R. Feldman, PhD, RN, FAAN, Editor

This quarterly is designed for professional nurses who perform leadership functions with clients, colleagues, health care institutions, and communities. It addresses the many facets of leadership through debate, interviews and thought-provoking current articles. This unique forum discusses the vital importance of nursing leadership in the public debates of health care reform.

NURSING
LEADERSHIP
FORUM

"A substantive journal for practicing nurse leaders. Solid content, timely, and a welcome source of relevant information."
—Dr. Maryann F. Fralic
Johns Hopkins University, School of Nursing

"No concept is talked about in these turbulent times more than 'leadership,' but often in very surface ways. Nursing Leadership Forum _provides a regular opportunity, by contrast, to have focused and extended discussion in this area."_
—Angela Barron McBride, PhD, RN, FAAN
Indiana University, School of Nursing

"...NLF consistently engages the reader in sharing an appealing vision of nursing leadership."
—Olga Maranjian Church, PhD, FAAN
University of Connecticut, School of Nursing

Sample Contents:

POINT/COUNTERPOINT

- Point: HIPAA Privacy and Primary Care Operations
- Counterpoint: HIPAA Impacts for Primary Care: Will the Burdens Outweigh the Benefits?

ARTICLES

- Keeping Codes Current: An Ethics Program to Support Nursing Practice
- Perceptions of First-Line Nurse Managers: What Competencies are Needed to Fulfill This Role?
- Medication Errors: A Bitter Pill

INDEXED / ABSTRACTED in: CINAHL, MEDLINE International Nursing Index, Social Services Abstracts, and Sociological Abstracts.

Volume 8 (2003-2004) • 4 issues • ISSN 1076-1632
Fall, Winter, Spring, Summer

536 Broadway, New York, NY 10012 • Telephone: 212-431-4370
Fax: 212-941-7842 • Order Toll-Free: 877-687-7476 • Order On-line: www.springerpub.com

Springer Publishing Company

Nursing and Health Policy Review – Journal –

Barbara K. Redman, PhD, RN, FAAN
and Ada K. Jacox, PhD, RN, FAAN, Editors

Nursing and Health Policy Review is a journal that promotes nursing's contribution to health policy on an institutional, local, national, and international level. It addresses the critical question: *How can nursing enter the mainstream of the ongoing health policy debate?* The purpose of the **Review** is to construct a conversation among nurses, policy makers, managers of health care institutions, economists, and other health professionals. It facilitates the thoughtful discourse necessary to promote and understand the importance of the nursing perspective in the complex, multidisciplinary world of health care.

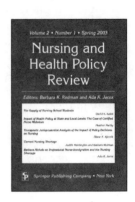

Sample Contents:

- Long-Term Health Care Policy for Elders: Now is the Time for Nursing Leadership, *Meridean L. Maas, Janet P. Specht, and Kathleen C. Buckwalter*

- Dr. Loretta Ford's Observation on Nursing's Past and Future, *Interview by Ada K. Jacox*

- Selective Attention in Health Policy and its Justification, *Barbara K. Redman and Ada K. Jacox*

- Response to David Mechanic and Susan Reinhard, *Shirley A. Smoyak*

- Role of the Government Chief Nurse in Policy and the Profession, *Frances A. Hughes*

- Sending for Nurses: Foreign Nurse Migration, 1965-2002, *Barbara L. Brush and Anne M. Berger*

- Hospital Downsizing: International Experiences and Perspectives, *Lynn Y. Unruh and Jacqueline Fowler Byers*

- Book Review, The Long Struggle: Nursing, Physician Control, and the Medical Monopoly, *Thetis M. Group and Joan I. Roberts, Reviewed by Barbara K. Redman*

Volume 2, 2003 • (2 Issues) • ISSN 1533-208X
Published 2 times per year: Spring, Fall

536 Broadway, New York, NY 10012 • Telephone: 212-431-4370
Fax: 212-941-7842 • Order Toll-Free: 877-687-7476
Order On-line: www.springerpub.com